BASIC MEDICAL TERMINOLOGY CONCEPTS

MARILYN WHITE WILSON

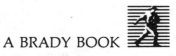

A BRADY BOOK

PRENTICE HALL BUILDING, Englewood Cliffs, New Jersey 07632

Library of Congress Cataloging-in-Publication Data

Wilson, Marilyn White
  Basic medical terminology concepts.

  Includes index.
    1. Medicine--Terminology. 2. Medicine--Terminology--
Problems, exercises, etc. I. Title. [DNLM:
1. Nomenclature. W 15 W751b]
R123.W48 1989   610'.14   88-19644
ISBN 0-89303-125-9

Editorial/production supervision and
  interior design: *Millicent Lambert*
Cover design: *Diane Saxe*
Manufacturing buyer: *Bob Anderson*

© 1989 by Prentice-Hall, Inc.
A Division of Simon & Schuster
Englewood Cliffs, New Jersey 07632

Printed in the United States of America
10 9 8 7 6 5 4 3

ISBN 0-89303-125-9

Prentice-Hall International (UK) Limited, *London*
Prentice-Hall of Australia Pty. Limited, *Sydney*
Prentice-Hall Canada Inc., *Toronto*
Prentice-Hall Hispanoamericana, S.A., *Mexico*
Prentice-Hall of India Private Limited, *New Delhi*
Prentice-Hall of Japan, Inc., *Tokyo*
Simon & Schuster Asia Pte. Ltd., *Singapore*
Editora Prentice-Hall do Brasil, Ltda., *Rio de Janeiro*

CONTENTS

PREFACE

Basic Medical Terminology Concepts introduces a system of medical word analysis that can be applied to the continual learning of new terminology, and includes prefixes, suffixes, and roots, with a heavy emphasis on the utilization of the newly learned "words" in a variety of exercise formats. Very basic anatomy is covered as well as an overview of the various specialties of the practice of medicine. The final chapter concentrates on putting to use all information garnered during the course through the application of this knowledge in defining actual medical reports. The completion of this text/workbook will provide familiarity with and knowledge of basic medical terms for those either in jobs requiring terminology or those wanting to learn the skills necessary for entry into medical fields, including transcription, insurance coding, and ward clerking. This volume utilizes a system of word analysis that can be applied to the continual learning of terminology in both clinical and research medicine.

This particular concept of learning medical terminology differs from the standard anatomy-physiology approach because of the emphasis on skills required by secretarial and support personnel. It is not intended to be a detailed anatomy and physiology text, since most support personnel and/or staff do not require an intricate knowledge of the names of each nerve in the hand or the names of each bone in the foot, for example. Instead, the focus is on on-the-job application as well as linguistic skills for both clerical and support personnel.

Occasionally one is fortunate enough to work for an individual who takes the time and has the patience to answer questions posed by a new employee. Such was the case with James D. O'Keefe, M.D., a physician in the San Antonio area, who answered questions and drew pictures for a neophyte medical secretary many, many years ago. Because of his care and concern, my curiosity was piqued and learning terminology became a thing of joy. He has my thanks forever. Several physicians and their staff, my family and friends, and in particular, Rose Belto, have my unending gratitude for their assistance and encouragement. The caring, interest, and willing help through the years by my daughter, Tamasyn, has been invaluable. My appreciation is boundless.

INTRODUCTION

Medical terminology is the tool required for the understanding, transscription, and pronunciation of the majority of not only medical terms, but words used in everyday conversation and reading. For example, *sub* is always defined as meaning **under** or **below,** whether you are referring to a submarine (under or below the ocean) or subcostal (under or below the rib); *tele* means **far away,** whether used in telescope (instrument for examining something far away) or telecardiograph (lines or drawings of the heart from far away); *mega* means **abnormally large,** as in megaphone (abnormally large sound or voice) or megacolon (abnormally large or very large colon).

Basic Medical Terminology Concepts is a system of word analysis for the study of terms and/or words related to any type of medicine or the medical practice. Medical terminology is used to describe all parts of the body in both the normal and abnormal state and includes all diseases and the diagnostic methods used in identifying diseases and their causes and treatments, whether surgical, medical, or a combination thereof. It also includes injuries and laboratory techniques as well as equipment used in the laboratory and in the rehabilitation of the patient. While the vocabulary is enormous (picked up a comprehensive medical dictionary lately?), many of the words use the same bits and pieces to be learned here. These bits and pieces are called prefixes, suffixes, and roots, or stem words, and are the building blocks of terminology. By using the proper combination, one can create a word

1

having either a very specific or ambiguous meaning, depending on the circumstances.

Many of the word pieces found in this text are ones already known. The brand name Magnavox means large (*magna*) voice (*vox*). Other examples include Chloraseptic—pathogens or toxins (*septic*), away (*a*), green (*chlor*), or something green that takes away or removes poisons (toxins) or germs. Noxzema comes from *nox* (night) plus *zema* (a drink). The name Listerine is taken from Lister, the man who founded anti-septic or **aseptic** surgery. Nyquil comes from *ny* (night) and *qui(e)* (resting). Aspirin comes from *aspi* (a shield) and *pyrin* (of fire). The word deodorant is formed by combining *de* (remove or away) and *odor* (scent or smell). The list goes on.

When using terminology, familiarity with the entire word, both alone and in its given context, is essential. Understanding what the word means ensures accurate transcription and translation. Students learn the exact meaning and spelling of words as well as correct pronunciation of each word (even though the person dictating the word may not always pronounce it correctly). This skill enables anyone to decipher the made-up words used by physicians, who may, at times, combine prefixes, suffixes, and root words to describe a particular situation exactly. Occasionally this new word will come into common usage through the publication of manuscripts by physicians.

Word definitions are learned through dexterity in breaking them into easily learned and understood components. As a rule, each word is made up of one or more stems and the attachment of the describing prefixes and/or suffixes, which add information to the root(s) by giving a full and complete description of the root word itself, stating how, when, where, or why things were done or happened.

Some encountered words will be of few syllables and therefore seem easy to break down. Do not let longer words put you off; they are often equally easy to understand, for by deciphering several word parts or sections, you can make an educated guess about their definition from their context, and thus find the words in a dictionary when proofreading.

Spelling of these words or pieces is of primary importance. The misunderstanding of a pronunciation, or the omission of a single letter, can change the meaning of a word or even reverse the meaning. A prime example of this is hyp*e*rtension (meaning high blood pressure) and hyp*o*tension (low blood pressure). Another common error occurs with words that sound alike: il*i*um is a bone in the pelvic area, part of the pelvic girdle; il*e*um is the last portion of small intestine. You must be able to distinguish these words by context.

While one can pick up an extensive medical vocabulary after a period of years in a medical environment, it is far easier to learn the lingo by memorizing the bits and pieces and being able to put them together.

The primary intent of this book is to enable anyone to see or hear any large medical word and then be able to break it down into familiar, easily defined, and understood components. Longer words are actually easier to define, because they have more syllables and more recognizable word pieces. Therefore, one can make an educated guess at the meaning of the unknown word pieces, or can define the word through its context. Pronunciation of any word is possible through the memorization of a few rules. These rules, like most, have many exceptions, but learning the rules will help.

The words in Chapter 3, Previewing Prefixes, Chapter 4, Zeroing in on Suffixes, and Chapter 5, Getting Down to Roots, are listed in their most commonly used divisions. These classifications do not mean that once a word part is pigeonholed as a prefix, it will always be found as the first syllable in a word or can never be used as either a suffix or root. These divisions merely serve as a method to facilitate systematic instruction, simplifying the learning process. Some words are used or found in just one system, but the majority are used in several systems as a descriptive word for a particular function of that system, be it an illness or problem relating to that system influenced by another system. Some words are used solely in the discussion of one biological system, but most words are used to describe the function, illness, or problems of multiple systems and their effects on one another.

There are several different exercises included. Some are just for fun; some take a lot of thought, and some (the crossword puzzles, for example) include words other than medical ones.

Making flash cards for the prefixes, suffixes, and roots is highly recommended as a study aid. Use different-colored cards for each set. The more these cards are used, the easier the words will become. These words are the building blocks, or components, used most often in a majority of frequently used medical words.

There are some areas that are not covered in great detail. Because laboratory equipment and surgical instruments are highly specialized, they are not dealt with here. Abbreviations are another topic not addressed in this text. All medical dictionaries list standard abbreviations;

each area of medicine has very specific and specialized abbreviations; moreover, some abbreviations are favored by only some physicians and in some geographic areas.

At the conclusion of this book, you will have a working knowledge of most medical words as well as the skill to learn new words found in specific work situations. The knowledge that a "five-dollar word" is nothing more than small bits or words whose meanings you already know should give you a great deal of self-confidence.

There is one primary rule to remember: If in doubt about the spelling of any word, look it up. Don't be afraid to ask questions. Inquiry is the best method of becoming proficient at any task.

SELF-DEFINING
WORDS

These words are in addition to the examples given in other chapters. They may be utilized—either orally or written on a blackboard—as examples of what students may already know but may not relate to medical terminology.

Word	Source A	Source B
taxidermist	taxi(s): arrangement	derm: skin (ist: one who)
telephone	tele: far away	phone: sound, voice
microscope	micro: small	scope, scopy: examine
phonograph	phono: sound, voice	graph: writing, lines
centipede	centi: hundred	ped(e): feet
aeroplane (airplane)	aero: air	plane: wanderer, rover
Frigidaire	frigid: cold	aire: air
transcontinental	trans: across	continental: pertaining to continent

Word	Source A	Source B
acrobat	acro: topmost, top, height	bat: one that walks, haunts
telegraph	tele: far away	graph: lines or drawings, write, writing
quadrangle	quad: four	angle: angle
bicycle	bi: two	cycle: circle, wheel
automobile	auto: self	mobile; move
platypus	platy: broad, flat	pus: foot
astronaut	astro: star	naut: ship, sail, sailor
antebellum	ante: before	bellum: the war (used word for Civil War)
prenatal	pre: before	natal: birth
absence	ab: away from	sence: presence
monorail	mono: one	rail: self-explanatory
amphibious	amphi: two, of two kinds	bio: life; ous: full of

PRETEST

Match the word parts in the left column with definitions in the right column.

Part A

_____	1. mit	a.	breath
_____	2. odes	b.	breathing
_____	3. ole	c.	constriction, compression
_____	4. otomy	d.	cutting, incision
_____	5. scopy	e.	disease
_____	6. ule	f.	dropping of an organ
_____	7. pathy	g.	education, child
_____	8. oda	h.	examine, observation
_____	9. rrhaphy	i.	form, resemblance, like
_____	10. stalsis	j.	giving birth to
_____	11. ology	k.	hard
_____	12. ptosis	l.	like, resemblance
_____	13. oid	m.	like, resemblance
_____	14. sclero	n.	opening into, communication between

_____	15.	oma	o. process/condition of, disease, act of
_____	16.	osis	p. sent, full of
_____	17.	phag	q. small
_____	18.	parous	r. small
_____	19.	pnea	s. spitting, saliva
_____	20.	sophy	t. study of, science of
_____	21.	spire	u. suture, repair
_____	22.	tropic	v. swallow, eating
_____	23.	stomy	w. tumor, growth
_____	24.	pedia	x. too few
_____	25.	penia	y. turning toward, tending to turn/change
_____	26.	ptysis	z. wisdom, art, skill

Part B

_____	27.	phobia	a. abnormal fear of, dread
_____	28.	taxis	b. anything formed
_____	29.	trophy	c. anything formed
_____	30.	plasm	d. arrangement
_____	31.	pod	e. blood vessel, vessel
_____	32.	ped	f. cell
_____	33.	plast	g. chest
_____	34.	osis	h. child, foot
_____	35.	tomy	i. clot
_____	36.	uria	j. cutting, incision
_____	37.	adeno	k. foot
_____	38.	vaso	l. fungus
_____	39.	cyto	m. gland
_____	40.	histo	n. in the urine
_____	41.	myo	o. liver
_____	42.	thoraco	p. marrow, spinal cord
_____	43.	procto	q. muscle
_____	44.	salpingo	r. nose

_____	45.	myelo	s.	nourishment
_____	46.	myco	t.	ovary
_____	47.	pyelo	u.	process, condition of, disease
_____	48.	rhino, naso	v.	rectum
_____	49.	oophoro	w.	renal pelvis, pelvis of kidney
_____	50.	thrombo	x.	skin
_____	51.	derma	y.	tissue
_____	52.	hepato	z.	tube

Part C

_____	53.	entero	a.	blood vessel
_____	54.	orchi	b.	bone
_____	55.	cardio	c.	breast
_____	56.	mast	d.	connective tissue
_____	57.	renal	e.	ear
_____	58.	gastro	f.	eye
_____	59.	oculo/ophthalmo	g.	fat
_____	60.	psyche	h.	heart
_____	61.	neuro	i.	intestine
_____	62.	arthro	j.	joint
_____	63.	angio	k.	kidney
_____	64.	costo	l.	lung, air
_____	65.	nephro	m.	mind
_____	66.	phlebo, ven(a, o)	n.	mucus
_____	67.	ot	o.	nerve
_____	68.	fibro	p.	pertaining to kidney
_____	69.	hystero	q.	rib
_____	70.	cysto	r.	sac, bladder
_____	71.	osteo	s.	stomach
_____	72.	muco	t.	testicle
_____	73.	lipo	u.	uterus
_____	74.	pneumo	v.	vein

Fill in the blanks.

75. Retrolingual means _____ the

   _____ .

76. Anesthesia means lack of _____ .

77. Mononeural means one _____ .

78. Hypotension means _____ pressure.

79. Polyuria means _____ urination.

80. Cyanosis means a _____ of being

   _____ .

81. Intravenous means _____ a

   _____ .

82. Excise means to _____ .

83. Malnutrition means nutrition that is _____ .

84. Glucogenic means _____ by
   sugar.

85. Macroencephaly means a large _____ .

86. Megacolon means a _____ that is

   _____ .

87. Necrophobia means an _____ of

   _____ .

88. Heterosexual means _____ .

89. Lipoderm is _____ skin.

90. Neuralgia means _____

in a _____ .

91. Hematemesis means _____ .

92. Pyogenic means _____ .

93. Endocarditis means _____ of

the _____ from within.

94. Cholelithiasis: condition of _____
in bladder (gallbladder).

95. Phagocytosis means a condition of _____

_____ .

96. Anodyne is _____ .

97. Microscope: an instrument to examine something _____

_____ .

98. Telescope: an instrument to examine something _____

_____ .

99. Atrophy is a lack of _____ .

100. Android means _____ man.

BODY AND DISEASE
SCIENCES
1

STUDY OF THE BODY

There are six primary branches of science that deal with the study of the body:

anatomy
physiology
pathology
embryology
histology
biology

Anatomy

This is the study of the structure of the body and the relationship of its parts.

Translated literally, the term anatomy means throughout *(ana)* and to cut *(tomy)* and is derived from the fact that human body structure is largely learned through dissection.

Physiology

This is the study of normal functions and activities of the body.

Physio refers to the relationship to nature and *logy* means the study of.

Pathology

This is the study of the changes caused by disease in the structure or functions of the body.

Patho means disease; this specialty deals primarily with tissue samples and organs removed either during surgery or **autopsy** (sometimes called **necropsy**), and through study, identifying the disease and/or pathogens present. The results provide the family and physician with a definitive diagnosis and often guide disease management.

Embryology

This is the study of body development from the **ovum** (female reproductive cell) after union with the **sperm** (male reproductive cell) through the second month after conception.

The **embryo** represents the developing human from one week after conception through the second month. After this stage, the developing human is referred to as a **fetus**.

Histology

This is the microscopic study of the minute (small) structure, composition, and function of normal cells and tissues. *Histo* means tissue.

Biology

This includes the study of all forms of life. *Bio* refers to life, and this discipline studies plant life and animal life, including the study of humans.

BIOLOGICAL STRUCTURE AND FUNCTIONS

All biological structures are composed of **cells**, which make up **tissues** (groups of cells similar in nature), which make up **organs** (groups of tissues working together to perform a specific function), which make up **systems** (combinations of organs for a specific purpose). This forms the basic framework for all medical disciplines and specialties.

BASIC SYSTEMS

A **basic system** is a combination of organs. The following are examples of systems.

Integumentary System

This system is composed of skin, which covers and protects the body and regulates body temperature, excretion, and sensation.

Skeletal System

This system encompasses all bones, which are the body framework. It provides support for the organs and furnishes places of attachment for muscles.

Muscular System

Muscles, which provide force for body motion and are attached to the skeletal system, make up this system.

Respiratory System

This system focuses on breathing and the lungs, which absorb oxygen from the air and provide it to the blood, and excrete carbon dioxide, releasing it from the body.

Cardiovascular System

The heart and blood vessels providing blood transport and nourishment to all body parts comprise this system.

Lymphatic System

Lymph is one of the three main types of body fluid (the others being blood and tissue fluid). It is a colorless, odorless fluid that circulates within the lymphatic system and consists primarily of water (95%) and components of blood plasma as well as containing *lymphocytes*. This system takes blood plasma as it seeps through capillary walls, to the tissues, where it becomes tissue fluid. It is then drained and collected by the lymphatic system (where it becomes lymph) and eventually is returned to the blood, where it becomes plasma once again. The system is responsible for the exchange of protein and fluid with the blood from body tissue, as well as protecting the body from *pathogens* (germs).

Gastrointestinal System

This system covers ingestion, digestion (from mouth to stomach) through the large and small intestines (which digest and absorb food), and excretion of waste material from the intestines through the rectum and anus.

Genitourinary System

This system includes two kidneys (which make urine), the bladder (for urine storage), ureters (which transport urine from the kidneys to the bladder), the urethra (which transports urine from the bladder to excretion) and, in the male, the prostate (which makes and transports male reproductive cells for species continuation) and male genitals. See MALE REPRODUCTIVE SYSTEM.

Nervous Systems and the Five Special Senses

All nerves, as well as the five special senses of touch, taste, smell, feeling, and hearing interact, giving the body and brain an awareness of environment and enabling them to react.

Endocrine System

All endocrine system glands produce *hormones*, secretions which are sent through the bloodstream and act as chemical messengers to all body organs, sending instructions for growth, sexual attributes and reproduction, mental status and personality traits, etc. These glands include the thyroid, parathyroid, adrenal, ovaries, and so on.

Reproductive System

The reproduction system provides the mechanics for **fertilization** (the union of germ cells, *ova* and *sperm*) and the production of sexual hormones through the **gonads** (sex glands: ovaries in women, testes in men).

Female reproductive system   This consists of the ovaries, Fallopian tubes, uterus, cervix, and so on, which produce sex hormones and provide facilities for reproduction. This system is treated by a *gyne*cologist (*gyne* means woman).

Male reproductive system   This consists of the external genitalia (penis, testes and scrotum), the accessory glands (prostate, seminal vesicles, and Cowper's glands), and the ducts leading from the prostate to the urethra. Since the male reproductive system is so closely tied to the genitourinary system (*genito* refers to genitals) through use of the urethra, urologists are the physicians who treat the male reproductive system.

BASIC MEDICAL DISCIPLINES AND SPECIALTIES

Anesthesiology

Anesthesia is the loss of *(an)* feeling or sensation *(esthesia)*. Artificial or anesthesiologist-induced anesthesia is produced by a number of agents capable of bringing about partial or complete loss of feeling, sensation, or consciousness, and is considered **local** (in a specific area) or **general** (the entire body).

This branch of medicine is concerned with the administration of anesthetics and the condition of the patient while under anesthesia until awakening. It includes all types of anesthesia; the personnel work in conjunction not only with surgery, but obstetrics and gynecology, orthopedics, medicine, and so on.

Biochemistry

This area studies chemical reactions occurring in living *(bio)* organisms.

Medicine

This is one of the largest specialties; there are many *internists* (specialists in internal organs) with subspecialities.

Internal medicine   This focuses on the treatment of diseases of the internal organs by a physician called an *internist.* Do not confuse this word with the term *intern*, which refers to a graduate medical student receiving training in a hospital prior to being licensed to practice medicine, or a *resident*, a physician in training immediately after completing an *internship* and learning a subspeciality in medicine or surgery.

Cardiology   This specialty is the study of *(ology)* diseases of the heart *(cardi)* and treatment of patients with these diseases.

Clinical epidemiology   *Epidemi* means among the people, or an epidemic. Epidemiology is the clinical study of factors that influence the frequency and distribution of infectious, contagious, or recurring diseases in humans.

Clinical pharmacology   *Pharma(c)* means drug. Clinical pharmacology is the study of drugs and the effects of these drugs on patients.

Dermatology   This refers to the study of diseases of the skin *(derma)*, along with treatment of those diseases.

Endocrinology   *Endo* translates to within; *crin* means separate. Endocrinology is devoted to the study of endocrine glands and their hormone secretions and the effect on patients because of the over- or underproduction of these hormones.

Gastroenterology   This is the study of diseases of the intestines *(enter)* and the stomach *(gastro)*, and allied treatment.

General and ambulatory medicine   This refers to the treatment of walking/able-to-walk *(ambul)* patients—in other words, those who are not confined to bed. See INTERNIST, FAMILY PRACTICE OR GENERAL PRACTICE.

Geriatrics/Gerontology   This is the study of the disease processes in aging humans. *Gera* means old age; *gero* or *geron* means old man.

Hematology   Hematology is the science dealing with the study of blood *(hema)*. Hematologists specialize in the diagnosis and treatment of blood diseases.

Histology   *Histo*, by definition, is tissue. In medicine, a histologist looks into causes of allergies and their effects on tissues—for example, swelling caused by the release of too many histamines, hence, treatment with antihistamines for allergies, stuffy noses, bee stings, and so on. See IMMUNO-ALLERGY.

Human genetics   *Gene* literally means origin or birth, and this branch deals with the phenomena of heredity and laws governing it. This field is divided into clinical genetics and biochemical genetics.

1.   **clinical genetics**   This refers to the study of genetic factors influencing occurrence of an inherited condition. Areas of study include chromosomal aberrations causing conditions such as Down's syndrome or mental retardation; diseases such as Huntington's chorea, which are passed down through a family; and immunogenetics, genetic aspects of antigens and antibodies; and reactions that have particular significance in organ transplantation.

2.   **biochemical genetics**   This area is concerned with both the chemical and physical nature of genes and the mechanism(s) by which they control development and maintenance of organisms. It has become the study of many specific diseases now known to be inherited, including sickle cell anemia (hereditary anemia), inborn errors of metabolism (*phenylketonuria* or PKU), and genetically determined variations of responses to certain drugs.

Infectious diseases   This specialty includes study of diseases caused by parasitic organism(s) and transmitted person-to-person or insect/animal-to-person via organism transfer, and includes communicable diseases spread by direct contact with the infectious agent causing it, either by contact with body excreta or discharges, indirect contact with objects (drinking glasses, toys, etc.), or other vectors, including mice, rats, dogs, cats, flies, bats, mosquitoes, ticks, and other creatures capable of transmitting disease. See CLINICAL EPIDEMIOLOGY.

Immunology-allergy   Immunology (*immuno* means safe, free, or immune) includes the study of resistance of the body to the effects of a harmful agent, such as pathogenic microorganisms or their poisons, and has several subdivisions. A histologist practices immunology-allergy, and looks into causes of allergies and their effects on tissues (e.g., swelling caused by the release of too many histidines, hence, treatment with antihistamines for allergies, stuffy noses, and bee stings). *Histo*, by definition, is tissue.

One of the most widely discussed areas today is the study of acquired immunologies (known as induced immunity), which result from antibodies not normally present in the blood. The field also includes active, cellular, humoral, natural, and passive immunology.

Allergists study abnormal and individual hypersensitivity to substances that are ordinarily harmless, including pollens, dust, and animal hair. This field also includes work with diseases produced by allergies, including hay fever, asthma, urticaria (hives), eczema, contact dermatitis, and anaphylactic shock, which is caused by a severe allergic reaction produced by foods (tomatoes, avocados), beverages (wine, alcohol, milk), insect bites (bees, mosquitoes) and plants (poison oak, ivy, and sumac).

Neurology (neuro, nerve)   This is the scientific study of the nervous system, including all functions and disorders.

Oncology (onkos, tumor)   Oncology is the science that studies tumors, and includes (but is not limited to) cancerous (malignant) tumors. Physicians specializing in cancer treatments are oncologists.

Pulmonary disease   This area is concerned with disease affecting the pulmonary *(pulmo,* lung) system, including breathing disorders and lung disease.

Renal disease or nephrology   This specialty is concerned with diseases pertaining to the kidney *(ren, nephro),* bladder, and so on. It is also known as **urology.** Nephrologists are kidney specialists and are frequently involved in transplant and dialysis procedures. See GENITOURINARY SYSTEM.

Rheumatology   Rheumatologists are concerned with diseases marked by pain in joints or muscles, or problems commonly called arthritis, osteoarthritis, bursitis, sciatica, and others.

Urology   See RENAL DISEASE.

Microbiology

This scientific area is concerned with minute *(micro)* living *(bio)* organisms, including (but not limited to) bacteria and molds. This specialty is usually found in a research setting.

Obstetrics and Gynecology

While obstetrics and gynecology are often paired, it isn't uncommon to find a physician practicing only gynecology. The word element *obstetri* means midwife, and *gyne* means woman.

Obstetrics   This specialty deals with pregnancy, labor, and delivery, as well as any attendant problems.

Gynecology   This area is devoted to treatment of the female genital tract. Gynecology literally means study of women. Gynecologists often treat their patients for any problems with the urinary tract as well.

These specialists may subspecialize in family planning, genetic counseling, and fertility/infertility problems.

Pathology

Pathology is the scientific study of alterations produced by disease *(patho):* these alterations are usually found in a laboratory or research setting. There are several subspecialties, divisions or areas of practice in this area.

Clinical pathology   This refers to pathology applied to clinical problem solution, especially utilizing laboratory methods to confirm clinical diagnoses.

Comparative pathology   Comparative pathology is pathology applied to human disease processes compared with those of lower animal species.

Experimental pathology   This includes the study of artificially induced pathologic processes.

Oral pathology   This is treatment of conditions resulting in or caused by inborn or functional changes in mouth structure.

Surgical pathology   This is study of diseased tissue accessible to operative intervention, or tissue removed from patients during surgery, and is the branch of pathology most people are familiar with.

Pediatrics

This branch of medicine is devoted to curing diseases of children, and is named from *pedia* or *ped*, for child or education, and *atrics*, meaning cure. Pediatricians practice well-baby or child care (regular checkups, routine immunizations, etc.) as well as caring for newborns and childhood illnesses. This branch includes several subspecialties, and it is not unusual to find any of the *medicine* subspecialties being pediatric subspecialties as well. These include (but are not limited to) allergy, cardiology, endocrinology, neurology, hematology, oncology, nephrology, gastroenterology, and infectious diseases. One field rapidly expanding is prenatal pediatrics, where diagnosis and treatment are performed on the unborn child or fetus. Neonatology is the science/art of diagnosis and treatment of the newborn infant, or **neonate**, up to four weeks of age.

Pharmacology

This area deals with all aspects of drugs *(pharm)*, not only in the lab and clinical (office, hospital, and home) settings, but also including pharmacists. Specialties include:

Clinical pharmacy   This is the area of the professional pharmacist, and includes proper preparation and compounding of medicines/drugs, as well as dispensing of medicines/drugs and medical supplies with a physician's prescription.

Clinical pharmacology   This term refers to bedside (hospital) or home treatment of patients, and pertains to (or is founded upon) actual observations and treatment of patients, including dosage adjustments of drugs for the patient's particular metabolism, body weight, and so on, as opposed to theoretical or experimental procedures with drugs (see PHARMACOLOGY). It may also involve controlled applications of experimental drugs for studies of effects, both good and bad, under the auspices of careful clinical studies.

Pharmacology   This is the theoretical or experimental aspect of drugs and actions/reactions on organisms, and so on. This is the primary research arm of drugs; it is often a vital component of new drug development.

Physical Medicine—Rehabilitation

This area is also called PMR, or physiatry, and uses various methods of physical therapy in disease treatment, including thermal (heat) therapy, massage, and manipulation of the limbs, working toward the goal of relieving stiffness and promotion of patient mobility. The discipline is also active in making braces and special shoes for specific orthopedic problems. The name is derived from *physic*, meaning physical or natural.

Psychiatry

This branch of medicine deals with the diagnosis, treatment, and prevention of mental disorders. It also covers child psychology, drug/chemical dependence, consultations and the best-known specialty, psychology.

Psychology   This is the scientific study of mental processes and behavior, including abnormal, analytic, clinical, criminal, in-depth and long-term psychoanalysis, experimental, genetic (development of the mind in individuals and with the evolution in the race), Gestalt, physiologic (facts taught in neurology to show relationships between mental and nerve-related), and social aspects of mental life.

Descriptive psychiatry   This specialty includes the study, observation, and external factors that can be seen, heard, or felt.

Dynamic psychiatry   This is the study of emotional processes, their origins, and underlying mental mechanisms.

Sociology

Sociology includes the scientific study of human society and of social relationships, organizations, and social change. It also deals with the principles or processes governing social phenomena. Although a social science and not a medical science, sociology can relate to the medical field in many ways, one being the coordination of prescribed diets for medical conditions (for example, diabetes and ulcers) with the cultural and ethnic backgrounds of patients.

Radiology

This medical science (*radio*, ray) deals with use of X-rays, radioactive substances, and other forms of radiation for diagnosis and treatment of diseases, and also includes nuclear medicine, which covers the effects of ionizing radiation, specialty diagnosis, and/or therapy using radioisotopes, and so on. This field is also the area of the radiation oncologist, who treat tumors by radiation or radioactive drugs (**chemotherapy**).

Surgery

This discipline treats disease primarily through operative procedures. Categories include cardiothoracic (heart/thorax, chest), otorhinolaryngology (*oto* = ear, *rhino* = nose, *laryngo* = larynx or throat) or ENT (ears, nose, and throat), general, plastic/reconstructive, neurosurgery, oral, urology, and orthopedic.

The foregoing are generalized descriptions of some specialties and subspecialties found in the medical field. They are by no means complete; all fields grow daily, as new or different areas open up through research and according to the needs of the world population. Each specialty has an experimental arm or area, carrying out laboratory and clinical research.

MEDICAL SPECIALTIES

Board-certified or **board certification** are terms used in referring to physicians who successfully complete specialized programs and testing in their particular field through hospital residencies, which take several years. This extensive training follows their graduation from medical school (receiving their M.D., or medical doctor, degree) and regular internship and residency. Board certification is peer recognition that they are well trained in their field. They are normally called a **fellow** or **diplomate,** and are required to keep abreast of new procedures and advances in their field. Some areas of specialty require periodic retesting, or recertification. The majority of the fields listed in the preceding section have their area of certification, and a board-certified physician usually has a string of initials following his or her name and M.D., such as F.A.C.S.—Fellow, American College of Surgeons; F.A.C.O.G.—Fellow, American College of Obstetrics and Gynecology; and F.A.C.C.—Fellow, American College of Cardiology. These designate which board or college the physician is a fellow or diplomate in (e.g., A.B.O.—American Board of Ophthalmology).

Allergy—Allergist

These are the specialty and specialist dealing with conditions such as hay fever, asthma, and sensitivities to various foods or insects.

Anesthesiology—Anesthesiologist

These refer to the specialty and specialist dealing with administration of anesthetics, whether administered by inhalation or injection.

Bacteriology—Bacteriologist

Bacteriology is the study, usually for diagnostic purposes, of infections/infectious agents (bacteria) in blood and body secretions. The bacteriologist is usually found in a research or laboratory environment.

Biology—Biologist

Biology is the study of life, usually at or below the cellular level. The biologist is usually found in either a research or laboratory environment.

Cardiovascular Disease—Cardiologist

Cardiovascular disease is disease of the heart and blood vessels. A cardiologist is usually an internist, or a physician specializing in internal medicine.

Dermatology—Dermatologist

These are the specialty and specialist dealing with treatment of skin diseases, including (but not limited to) acne, rashes, and moles. The dermatologist also treats other skin problems, like brown recluse spider bites.

Family Practice—Family Practitioner

This area was once called a **general practice:** the old-time family doctor was known as a **G.P.** There is now board certification for family practice, which requires a specified period of residency.

Hematology—Hematologist

Hematology is the study of blood and its abnormalities. The hematologist deals with diagnostics and structures treatments in conjunction with the referring or primary-care physician.

Gastroenterology—Gastroenterologist

This area (sometimes known as GI, from gastrointestinal) deals with diseases of the stomach and/or intestines. A physician in this field is usually an internist, as well.

General Practice—General Practitioner

These refer to the G.P., or family doctor. This is not a board-certified specialty.

Gerontology—Gerontologist

This is the specialty and specialist in diseases and problems of aging populations.

Gynecology—Gynecologist

This is the area of specialization for diseases of the female reproductive system.

Industrial Medicine

This is a specialty concerned primarily with protection against occupational hazards, such as poisoning by lead or other chemical exposure, and treatment of these exposures.

Internal Medicine—Internist

This specialty and specialist are concerned with diseases of organs and organ systems, dealing primarily with diagnosis and nonsurgical intervention of diseases and nonsurgical treatment of adults in general. It is not unusual for an internist to have a subspecialty and to practice primarily in that area—for example, in cardiology, gastroenterology, and so on.

Neurology—Neurologist

The focus of this area is on diseases of or relating to the nervous system.

Neurosurgery—Neurosurgeon

This is the specialty and specialist concerned with surgical intervention for diseases or trauma to the brain, spinal cord, and/or nerves.

Obstetrics—Obstetrician

This specialty is dedicated to the treatment of pregnant females through delivery and during the postpartum period. Some also specialize in fertility problems.

Oncology—Oncologist

These refer to the specialty and specialist in malignant neoplasm or tumor treatments.

Ophthalmology—Ophthalmologist

This area is concerned with diseases of the eye and associated structures. These physicians also write prescriptions for eyeglasses.

Orthopedics—Orthopedist

This is the specialty and specialist concerned with treatment of bones, joints, and muscles, primarily involving trauma to those areas.

Otorhinolaryngology—Otorhinolaryngologist

These refer to the treatment of diseases in the ear, nose, and throat (hence the more common ENT).

Pathology—Pathologist

These are concerned with the study of abnormal tissues that have been removed from the body, either for diagnostics or after surgery.

Some subspecialties are criminal pathology, also known as *forensic pathology*, and *clinical pathology*, the area concerned with examination of blood, secretions, and excretions by chemical and/or microscopic methods.

Pediatrics—Pediatrician

These are the specialty and specialist in (but not limited to) infants and children and their problems. Some pediatricians treat patients through the teens, and some now treat babies before they are born. There are also pediatricians who specialize in any of the other areas, but dealing specifically with the effects and treatment for children, as in a pediatric cardiologist, pediatric oncologist, and so on. Several diseases found in both adults and children are treated in a completely different manner in the very young or very old.

Plastic Surgery—Plastic Surgeon

These pursue the reconstruction of any part of the body that has been damaged either by disease, trauma, or age. Plastic surgery includes both corrective and cosmetic surgery.

Proctology—Proctologist

These deal with diseases of the rectum, colon, and related surgeries. Proctology is sometimes a subspeciality of a gastroenterologist.

Psychiatry—Psychiatrist

This specialist treats diseases of the mind. Some areas also treat the associated problems of chemical and substance abuse and its effect on behavior.

Public Health

This field is concerned primarily with sanitation and the prevention and control of epidemic diseases, and an investigative tracking of epidemic causes. A prime example is the Centers for Disease Control, in Altanta, Georgia, which focus on investigations of disease outbreaks, or **pandemics**, throughout the United States. Clinical epidemiologists frequently work in public health, and the discipline of infectious diseases is included in this cateogry.

Radiology—Radiologist

This area uses X-rays for diagnostic purposes and for treatment of various diseases. Nuclear medicine deals with the use of radioactive substances for diagnosis and treatment of various diseases.

Surgery—Surgeon

This branch of medicine deals with the manual and operative procedures for the correction of deformities and defects, whether caused by genetics, disease, or trauma, and treatment for suffering from disease and for the prolongation of life. Some of the surgical subspecialties are:

Oral surgeon   This person deals with surgical treatment of diseases of the mouth. Note: Sometimes, but not always, oral surgeons are also dentists.

Orthopedic surgeon   This person specializes in surgical treatment of injuries and deformities of the skeletal, as well as muscular, systems.

Thoracic surgeon   One who is concerned with surgical treatment of diseases of the chest and organs found therein.

Urology—Urologist

This is the specialty and specialist dealing with treatment of disorders of the entire urinary tract of both men and women, as well as the genital organs and fertility problems in the male.

1. MEDICAL DISCIPLINES COMPLETION EXERCISE

Fill in the blank with the word that most correctly completes the sentence.

1. Heart disease is studied by a _____ .

2. Chemical reactions occurring in living organisms are studied in

    _____ .

3. The study of diseases of the intestines and stomach is called

    _____ .

4. One of the largest specialties, covering treatment of most disease

    processes, is _____ .

5. The area that studies skin disease is _____

    _____ .

6. Clinical pharmacology studies effects of _____

    _____ on patients.

7. The loss of feeling or sensation is _____ .

8. Hormonal problems are studied by _____ .

9. One treating pregnancy and childbirth is called an _____

    _____ .

10. Blood diseases are treated by the specialty of _____

    _____ .

11. The branch of medicine dealing with all aspects of drugs is

    _____ .

12. Inherited diseases are studied by a _____

    _____ .

13. Infectious diseases are diseases caused by organisms or by an

    _____ .

14. The branch of medicine dealing with the removal of any tissue is

    _____ .

15. The specialty dealing with the overall treatment of children is

    _____ .

16. Resistance of the body to the effects of a harmful agent is treated by

    _____ .

17. Hypersensitivity to an agent is studied by an _____

    _____ .

18. Minute living organisms are studied by an _____

    _____ .

19. Frequency and distribution of infectious diseases are studied by an

    _____ .

20. Breathing problems are studied by someone specializing in

    _____ diseases.

21. The specialty concerned with kidneys and bladders is _____

_____ .

22. A graduate medical student completing his training in a hospital

setting is called an _____ or

_____ .

23. Rheumatologists work with diseases causing pain in _____

_____ or _____ .

24. A specialist in women's diseases is a _____

25. Nuclear medicine is a branch of medicine dealing with nonionizing

_____ .

26. The scientific study of alterations produced by diseases is called

_____ .

27. Aging patients are often treated by one in the field of _____

_____ .

28. The branch of medicine dealing with X-rays and diagnosis from

them is called _____ .

29. The scientific study of mental processes and behavior is

_____ .

30. One filling a prescription to the doctor's specifications is a

_____ .

2. MEDICAL DISCIPLINES IDENTIFICATION EXERCISE

List and define the six branches of science.

1. _____

   _____

2. _____

   _____

3. _____

   _____

4. _____

   _____

5. _____

   _____

6. _____

   _____

Define the following terms and use them in words learned in the fore-going sections.

7. patho _____

8. bio _____

9. uro _____

10. ortho _____

11. physio _____

12. ped (Greek) _____

13. ped (Latin) _____

14. histo _____

15. oto _____

16. derm _____

17. gynec _____

18. ophthalmo _____

19. psych _____

20. geri _____

Name the branch of medicine and type of physician treating the following organs and systems.

21. urinary tract _____

22. heart _____

23. skin _____

24. female genital tract _____

25. endocrine glands _____

26. internal organs _____

27. X-ray interpretation _____

28. diseases of the mind _____

29. ears _____

30. backache _____

31. male infertility _____

32. larynx, pharynx, nasopharynx, and tracheobronchial tree ____

     _____

33. radiation, ionizing radiation effects or treatment with nonioniz-

     ing radiation _____

     _____

34. effects of space exploration on astronauts _____

35. physical therapy in disease treatment _____

36. male urinary system _____

37. broken bones _____

38. problems with the gastrointestinal tract _____

39. abnormal blood cells _____

Name the specialty that treats the following conditions.

40. deformed foot _____

41. brain tumor _____

42. face lift _____

43. surgical removal of a wisdom tooth _____

44. sleep prior to surgery _____

45. wound to the eyeball _____

46. partial paralysis or muscle atrophy _____

47. astronauts at NASA _____

48. injury incurred while at work _____

49. heart attack _____

50. hormonal imbalance _____

3. MEDICAL DISCIPLINES AND SPECIALTIES PUZZLE

ACROSS

2. Orthopedic specialty
5. Study of tumors
11. Study of
15. Make a mistake
17. Top of bikini
18. Before
19. Woodwind instrument
20. Kidney specialist
25. Related
27. Gastroenterologist
28. Unmarried lady
29. Part
30. Animal covering
31. Throat specialist
35. X-ray specialty
39. Path
41. Emote
42. Since, because
43. Pertaining to the anus
44. East Germany, (abbr.)
45. Female specialist
49. Large country homes
52. Knock out
54. A native of
56. Railroads (abbr.)
57. Skip
58. Bear sound
59. Otologist's specialty
62. Egyptian sun god

63. Disease alteration study
67. Enthusiasm
69. Rhode Island (abbr.)
70. Old horse
72. Immigration & Naturalization Service (abbr.)
73. Pertaining to skin
77. Extraterrestrial
79. Sweet _____
80. Half of English "bye"
82. Divorce capital
83. Robert E. _____
84. Domination
87. Side sheltered from wind
90. Do not
92. Additionally
93. Commercial
94. Eye specialist
98a. Manned
102. Opposite of yes
103. Koala bear (abbr.)
104. Noise of disgust
105. _____ Stanley Gardner
106. Otorhinolaryngologist (abbr.)
107. Alcoholics Anonymous (abbr.)
108. Agreement answer
110. Aft
113. Banish
114. Seethe

117. Spanish yes
118. Musical syllable
119. Carried
122. Tyke
123. Within
125. Theater box
126. Cher's first
128. Study of tissue
131. Los Angeles (abbr.)
133. Petrochemical product
134. District attorney (abbr.)
135. Obstetrician
136. Ophthalmologist specialty
138. Record
139. High card
140. Ethical
141. A long time _____
142. Nickname for Edward
143. Pertaining to the ear
144. Frosting
145. Room mother (abbr.)
147. General Electric
148. Flourish
150. Element
153. American Airlines (abbr.)
154. Copious
155. Laboratories, in short
157. Story
159. Medicine specialist

163. Death notices
165. Additional
167. Beside
168. Pose
169. Gynecologist (abbr.)
171. Prior to
172. Divides
173. Mind doctor
174. Protein source
175. Exist

DOWN

1. Nerve
2. Study of Life
3. New
4. Unit of energy
6. Spiral
7. Pound (abbr.)
8. Spree
9. Yield
10. Fiddler while Rome burned
11. Superman's Lane
12. Relating to childbirth
13. More than one go
14. Archaic you

3. (CONTINUED)

16. Fissure
18. Referring to rectum/anus
21. Portrayal
22. Appendage
23. Healer who cuts/removes
24. Platter
25. Reaction
26. Capture
28. Fine rain
32. Fume
33. Lettuce and Tomato (abbr.)
34. What a GI man is
35. Evaluate
36. Takes away from (prefix)
37. Baby's first syllable
38. Category
40. Not out
46. Sob
47. Mouth
48. Component
49. Chorus for Old MacDonald
50. Get a hold of
51. Imbibe
53. Where a surgeon works
54. He, she, or _____
55. Slender
60. One who puts you to sleep

61. Royal advisor (abbr.)
64. Study of body structure
65. Landing ship (abbr.)
66. Lemon – – –
67. Specialist
68. Aches
71. Old-age specialist
74. One who studies glands
75. Geriatric
76. Those born in August
78. Half a ballet skirt
79. Child specialist
81. Pie _____ mode
85. Tra _ la
86. Old Testament (abbr.)
88. Animal related to a moose
89. Study of embryo
91. Old sailor
95. Study of tissue
96. Hawaiian dance
97. Rent
98. Good Housekeeping (abbr.)
99. Throw
100. _ Fi Fo Fum, I smell . . .
101. Feared
107. While
109. Spanish for this

111. Ear specialists
112. Study of the heart
115. European Theater of Operations (abbr.)
116. Month after April
120. Automation
121. After DDD
124. Two
127. Form of no
128. Laugh
129. Part of a min.
130. Pathogen
132. Exist
137. Poetic, persons
146. Miraculous food
149. Part of a cry
151. Those who look
152. Female horse over two years
153. Competences
156. Part of a skeleton
158. Rhinologist specialty
160. Oto
161. Emergency signal
162. First part of a sneeze
163. Japanese sash
164. Hawaii hula skirt leaf
166. Rooster's companion
170. Your brother (abbr.)

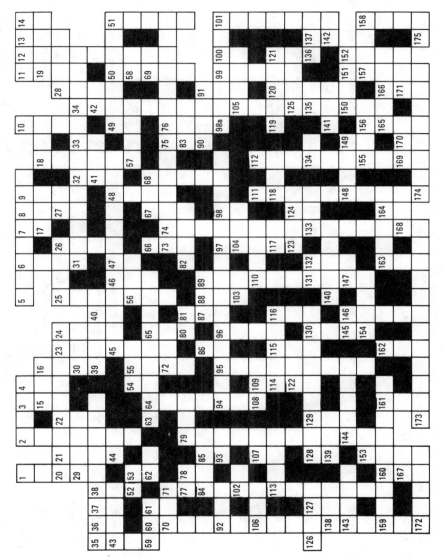

3. MEDICAL DISCIPLINES AND SPECIALTIES PUZZLE

39

4. SPECIALISTS AND THEIR SPECIALTIES PUZZLE

ACROSS

2. Neoplasm specialty
5. Takes pictures in the dark
10. Treatment
11. Heart specialist
15. Oxygen _____
17. Take out (abbr.)
18. Common name for intestine
20. Specialist for women only
26. Kidney specialist
29. R2D2
30. Found in an atlas
32. Louisiana (abbr.)
33. Cleopatra's "friend"
34. Specialty of disease alterations
36. Leave
37. Lisper's "thing"
41. Hematologist's specialty
42. Overstretch
43. Hormone specialist's field
45. Taken in midafternoon
46. Otologist's field
47. Physician of Internal medicine
48. A clue
52. Used in grocery store
53. They care for eyes
57. Long distance (abbr.)
58. It's a _____
59. Field of students of the mind
61. Ripped

63. Study of life
65. Camping items
66. Neurologist's field
69. Its bite sends you to an allergist
70. Catcher's glove
71. Allergists study this
73. What tape does
76. M.D.'s organization
77. Proctologist's field
78. Remover of tissue

DOWN

1. Concern and consideration
2. Neoplasm specialty
3. Flower garland
4. Rhinologist's specialty
5. Balance
6. Who takes care of your teeth?
7. Area for a chest surgeon
8. Doctor using operative procedures
9. What some have to a bee sting
12. Something to sweep dust under
13. Nickname for a family doctor
14. Those who study life
16. Run in a hurry
19. Pediatrician's patient
21. Shy
22. Obstetrician?
23. Means "ear"

24. Practitioner of internal medicine
25. Take care of
27. Young boy
28. Fuel for an automobile
31. He uses a proctoscope
34. _____ and needles
35. Study of body structure
38. Not out
39. Opposite of stop
40. Male fertility doctor
44. Specialty of doctor for older people
46. Black
48. Old Testament pronoun
49. Impersonal pronoun
50. Study normal functions
51. Sick
54. He's a physician
55. Your male child
56. Drug dispensary
60. Red skin
62. In a hurry
64. Orthopedics area
67. Vigor
68. Estimated time arrival
72. Desire
74. "_____ for the Tummy"
75. I am (contraction)

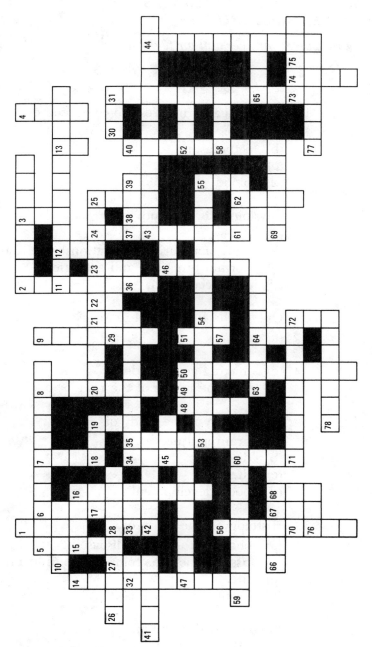

4. SPECIALISTS AND THEIR SPECIALTIES PUZZLE

5. BODY AND DISEASE SCIENCES
MULTIPLE CHOICE EXERCISE

Select the correct answer and write the letter of your choice in the space provided.

_____   1.   All medical structures are composed of
(a)   cells.
(b)   ectoplasm.
(c)   bones.
(d)   blood.

_____   2.   Physiology is the study of
(a)   disease.
(b)   body structure and relationship of parts.
(c)   normal functions and activities.
(d)   advanced math.

_____   3.   One of the five special senses is
(a)   ESP.
(b)   touch.
(c)   making good grades
(d)   to come in out of the rain.

_____   4.   Embryology is the study of
(a)   brain and nerves.
(b)   disease.
(c)   life.
(d)   body development.

_____   5.   Histology is the study of
(a)   changes caused by disease.
(b)   tissue structure, composition, and function.
(c)   life.
(d)   events prior to 1960.

_____   6.   Biology is the study of
(a)   plants and animals after death.
(b)   all forms of life.

(c) babies before they are born.
(d) none of the above.

_____   7. The integumentary system is made up of
(a) Juicy Fruit.
(b) papayas.
(c) gums beneath teeth.
(d) none of the above.

_____   8. A gynecologist
(a) takes care of babies.
(b) takes care of old men.
(c) takes care of women.
(d) takes care of teenagers.

_____   9. An anesthesiologist makes you
(a) have good circulation.
(b) pass your physical examination.
(c) feel no pain.
(d) none of the above.

_____   10. Disease processes in aging humans are studied by
(a) gerontologists.
(b) gastroenterologists.
(c) geneticists.
(d) pathologists.

_____   11. The respiratory system includes
(a) lungs.
(b) oxygen.
(c) carbon dioxide.
(d) the heart.

_____   12. Anatomy is the study of
(a) life.
(b) body structure and relationship of parts.
(c) normal functions and activities.
(d) disease.

_____ 13. The intestines are found in the
      (a) female reproductive system.
      (b) nervous system.
      (c) gastrointestinal system.
      (d) skeletal system.

_____ 14. The skeletal system is made up of
      (a) bones.
      (b) papier-mâché.
      (c) organs.
      (d) all of the above.

_____ 15. The urethra is found in which system?
      (a) genitourinary
      (b) integumentary
      (c) cardiovascular
      (d) none of the above

_____ 16. Hormones are produced by the
      (a) lymphatic system.
      (b) integumentary system.
      (c) skeletal system
      (d) endocrine system.

_____ 17. An allergy is
      (a) a hypersensitivity to something.
      (b) a hyposensitivity to something.
      (c) influenza.
      (d) a heart attack.

_____ 18. The Fallopian tubes are found in which system?
      (a) female reproductive
      (b) genitourinary
      (c) cardiovascular
      (d) muscular

_____ 19. All medical structures are composed of
      (a) cells.
      (b) ectoplasm.
      (c) bones.
      (d) blood.

_____ 20. Heart disease is treated by a(n)
      (a) endocrinologist.
      (b) gynecologist.
      (c) histologist.
      (d) cardiologist.

_____ 21. Pathology is the study of
      (a) disease.
      (b) normal cells and tissues.
      (c) life.
      (d) body development.

_____ 22. Children are taken care of by
      (a) gynecologists.
      (b) podiatrists.
      (c) pediatricians.
      (d) pathologists.

_____ 23. Endocrinology is the study of
      (a) the inside of the brain.
      (b) bones.
      (c) vessels and their fluids.
      (d) glands and hormone secretions.

_____ 24. Hematology is the study of
      (a) serum.
      (b) blood.
      (c) urine.
      (d) spinal fluid.

_____ 25. Genetics are
      (a) Levi's.
      (b) blind spots in the eye.
      (c) building blocks of life, or genes.
      (d) none of the above.

_____ 26. The cardiovascular system provides
      (a) electrocardiograms.
      (b) romantic novels.
      (c) pacemakers.
      (d) blood transport and nourishment.

_____ 27. For a broken bone you would see a
    (a)   plastic surgeon.
    (b)   orthopedist.
    (c)   anesthesiologist.
    (d)   gynecologist.

_____ 28. X-rays are interpreted by
    (a)   anesthesiologists.
    (b)   podiatrists.
    (c)   radiologists.
    (d)   psychiatrists.

_____ 29. A G.P. is
    (a)   a good person.
    (b)   a general pediatrician.
    (c)   a general practitioner.
    (d)   none of the above.

_____ 30. Psychiatry works with disorders of the
    (a)   mind.
    (b)   body.
    (c)   soul.
    (d)   brain.

PRONOUNCING AND SPELLING
MEDICAL TERMS

2

Medical terms often seem hard to pronounce, especially when they are seen in print but have never been heard or spoken. Through the study of prefixes, suffixes, and roots, and by careful pronunciation of each word piece as you learn it, your pronunciation will improve daily and your spelling skills will be enhanced. What follows are some rules and/or shortcuts that may be helpful. When reviewing the examples given, write in words that are in your current vocabulary that use the same rules. These will assist you in remembering the rules.

CONSONANTS

Ch   This sounds like *k* in **chromatin**, **chronic**, and **pachyderma**, unless the word is not Greek-based. The derivative of the word will be listed in the medical dictionary.

Ps   You only hear and pronounce the *s*, as in the words **psychiatry** and **psychology**.

Pn   Only the *n* sound is heard, as in **pneumonia**.

C and G   These are given the soft sounds of *s* and *j*, respectively, before *e*, *i*, and *y* in words of both Greek and Latin origin, as in **cycle**, **cytoplasm**, **giant**, and **generic**.

C and G   The letters *c* and *g* have harsh sounds before other letters, as in **cast**, **cardiac**, **gastric**, and **gonad**.

VOWELS

All vowels are pronounced, either with a long or short sound. When a vowel is at the end of a word (unless it is an *a*), it is pronounced with a long sound. The *a* is short, as in *uh*, in words like **amnesia**, **anoxia**, **carcinoma**, **dyspepsia**, **dysuria**, **edema**, and **hematuria**.

If there is a vowel in the last syllable of a word, the pronunciation is short, as in **antibiotic**, except *es*, which is pronounced like *ease*, as in **caries** and **herpes**.

Ae and oe   These are normally pronounced *ee*, as in **fasciae**.

Ai   This is pronounced with a short *a*, as in **ainhum** (an hum) or **aichmophobia** (ak mo fo be ah).

Au   The *au* combination is pronounced as in **August**.

Eu   The *eu* combination sounds like a hard *u*, as in **euthanasia**.

Ei   The *ei* is pronounced as a long *i*, as in **eidoptometry**.

E and es   The *e* and *es* are used when forming the final letter or letters of a word; they are often pronounced as a separate syllable, as in **rete** (ree tee) and **herpes** (her peez).

I   This is used at the end of a word to form a plural, and is pronounced as a long *i*, as in **alveoli**, **glomeruli**, and **fasciculi**.

Oe   Normally pronounced as a long *e*, as in **foetal** (British spelling of **fetal**).

FORMING PLURALS

The addition of an *s* or *es* forms the plural for most English words. However, in Greek and Latin (which are the basis for most medical words), a plural may be designated by changing the endings as follows:

. . .*ae*   A word that ends in *a* in the singular form may end in *ae* in the plural: **fasciae** (singular, *fascia*);

. . .*ata*   A word that ends in *a* in the singular form may end in *ata* in the plural: **adenomata** (singular, *adenoma*);

. . .*ia*   A word that ends in *ium* in the singular form may end in *ia* in the plural: **crania** (singular, *cranium*);
NOTE: *ia* is also a word element for a state or condition of, or disease, such as in **anesthesia.**

. . .*i*   When the singular form of a word ends in *us*, the plural form is made by dropping the *us* and adding an *i:* **glomeruli** (singular, *glomerulus*).

SPELLING RULES

All of the aforementioned rules for pronunciation and the formation of plurals are necessary for proper spelling, but it is essential that you consult a medical dictionary if you are not sure. In medical terminology, there are numerous exceptions to the rules. Proper pronunciation of the terms will enable you to spell them easily and more accurately.

Phonetic spelling has no place in medicine, because a misspelled word may give a completely incorrect meaning to a diagnosis. Furthermore, terms are sometimes pronounced alike but spelled differently, meaning totally different things. For example, **ileum** is a part of the intestinal tract, but **ilium** is a pelvic bone.

Overall, the primary rule is: *When in doubt, look it up.*

PREVIEWING *PREFIXES*

3

A **prefix** is, by definition, one or more letters or syllables placed at the beginning of a word to illustrate its significance; it modifies, changes, or enhances the root word or stem. Several of the listed prefixes will be familiar. In the word example, draw a slash between the prefix and the remainder of the word to visualize each word as composed of several small pieces; for example, tachycardia: tachy/cardia.

LOCATIONS

Prefix	Meaning	Word Example
ad	near to, near, toward	adrenal
ec, ecto	on the outside	ectoderm
endo	inner, inside, within	endoderm
epi	upon	epidermis
ex	outside, away	excise
extra	outside of	extracellular
inter	between	intercostal
intra	within	intravenous
meso	middle	mesoderm
para	beside, near, beyond, apart from	paramedian

LOCATIONS

Prefix	Meaning	Word Example
peri	around	periotic
retro	behind	retrosternal
retro	located behind	retrolingual
sub	under	subcutaneous, subdermal
super	above	superego
supra	above	supralumbar

TIME

Prefix	Meaning	Word Example
ante	before	antepartum
neo	new	neonatal
post	after	postmortem
pre	before	prefix, prenatal

NEGATION

Prefix	Meaning	Word Example
a, ab	from, away	abnormal
a, an	without	anesthesia
abs	from, away	absence
anti	against	antidote, antipyretic
de	remove, from	dehydrate

NUMBERS: AMOUNT OR COMPARISON

Prefix	Meaning	Word Example
mono	one, single	mononeural
uni	one, single,	uniform
bi, di	two, double	bicuspid, dissect
duo	two, double	duodenoduodenostomy
tri	three, triple	triangle
tetra	four	tetraplegia

NUMBERS: AMOUNT OR COMPARISON

Prefix	Meaning	Word Example
quadr	four	quadruped, quadriplegia, quadrantanopia
brady	slow	bradycardia
hemi	half	hemiplegia
hyper	too much, over, high	hypertension
hypo	too little, under, low	hypoglycemia
multi	many	multicellular
poly	many, much	polyuria
semi	partly, about half	semiconscious
tachy	fast	tachycardia

COLORS

Prefix	Meaning	Word Example
alb	white	albumin, albino
chloro	green	chlorophyll
chro	color	chromatic
cyano	blue	cyanosis, cyanotic
erythro	red	erythrocyte
leuco	white	leucocyte
leuko	white	leukocyte
lute	yellow	luteum (corpus luteum)
melan	black	melanoma

POSITIONS

Prefix	Meaning	Word Example
ambi	both	ambidextrous
amphi	about, both sides	amphibious
antero	in front	anterolateral
dextro	right	dextromanual
di	across	diameter
latero	to the side of	lateroversion

POSITIONS

Prefix	Meaning	Word Example
levo	left	levorotation
medio	middle	mediotarsal
opistho	backward, behind	opisthotic
postero	behind	posteromedial
trans	across	transverse

SIZE

Prefix	Meaning	Word Example
macro	abnormally large or big	macroencephaly
lepto	thin	leptodermic
mega	large (very, exceptionally)	megacolon
micro	very or abnormally small	microscope

MISCELLANEOUS

Prefix	Meaning	Word Example
acro	top, extremity, height	acrophobia
aero	air	aerocele
andro	man	android
bio	life	biology
crypt	hidden	cryptorchidism
dys	difficult, painful	dysuria
etio	cause	etiology
febr	fever	febrile
gluc, gluco	sweet, sugar	glucogenic
glyc, glyco	sweet, sugar	glycemia
gyne	woman	gynecology
hetero	different	heterosexual
hydro	water	hydrocephalus
lipo	fat	lipoderm
mal	bad	malnutrition
narc	sleep	narcotic

MISCELLANEOUS

Prefix	Meaning	Word Example
necro	death	necrophobia
noct	night	noctambulism
ortho	straight	orthodontist
pan	all	panacea
path	disease	pathology
pyo	pus	pyogenic
pyro	fever, fire	pyrogen, pyromaniac
tele	faraway, at a distance	telecardiograph

POSITIONS AND LOCATIONS

Word	Meaning
anterior	(*antero*, front) pertaining to front of body
caudal	pertaining to lower part of spinal column
cavity	any hollow space
cephalad	toward the head
cranial	pertaining to head or skull
distal	farthest from point of attachment
dorsal	pertaining to the back of body
external	outside
inferior	below
internal	inside
lateral	(*latero*, side) pertaining to side of body
medial	(*medio*, middle) toward the midline
parietal	pertaining to wall of a structure
peripheral	near the surface
posterior	(*postero*, back) pertaining to the back of body
prone	lying on face
proximal	nearest point of attachment
superior	above
supine	lying on back
ventral	pertaining to the front of the body
visceral	pertaining to structures found inside the body

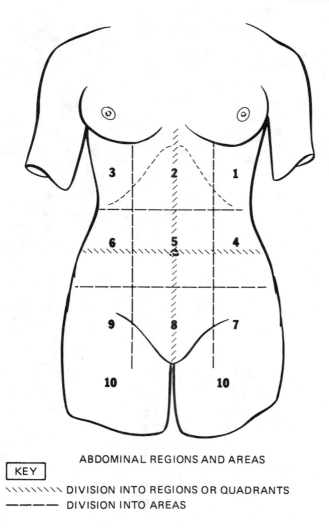

ABDOMINAL REGIONS AND AREAS

KEY

\\\\\\\\ DIVISION INTO REGIONS OR QUADRANTS

———— DIVISION INTO AREAS

ABDOMINAL REGIONS

The abdomen is divided into four parts or quarters, also known as **regions** or **quadrants**. Right and left refer to patient's right and left. They are:

    Right upper quadrant
    Right lower quadrant
    Left upper quadrant
    Left lower quadrant

These regions are broken down into the following areas:

1. Left hypochondriac
2. Epigastric
3. Right hypochondriac
4. Left lumbar
5. Umbilical
6. Right lumbar
7. Left inguinal or left iliac
8. Hypogastric or pubic
9. Right inguinal or right iliac
10. Femoral

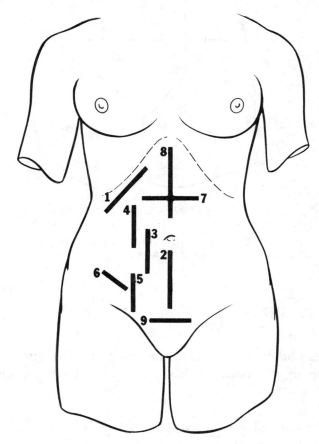

BASIC SURGICAL INCISIONS

BASIC SURGICAL INCISIONS

What follows is a list of basic incisions. These incisions are ones most commonly used in abdominal surgeries. They appear on the drawing as numbers by a line indicating each incision.

1. Subcostal
2. Midline
3. Mid-rectus
4. Upper right rectus
5. Lower right rectus
6. McBurney's
7. Transverse
8. Paramedian
9. Suprapubic

POSITIONS FOR SURGERY AND EXAMINATION

The more common positions for either surgery or examination are included.

Dorsal or supine   Lying on back, legs straight, head in line with body; arms alongside body, palms down.

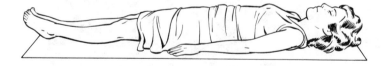

Dorsal recumbent   Lying on back, head in line with body, knees bent at 45° angle; arms alongside body, palms down.

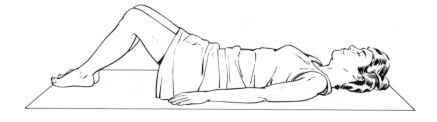

Trendelenberg   On back with knees bent over lower break of examination table; arms alongside body, palms down, head and knees lower than middle of body, *or* legs/feet elevated, body prone (as depicted in figure).

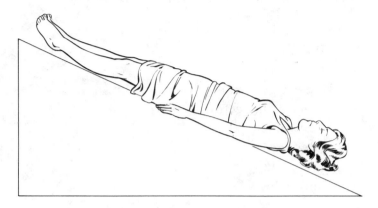

Dorsal lithotomy   On back, knees raised well over buttocks, arms crossed over chest, feet in stirrups, flexed, and rotated outward.

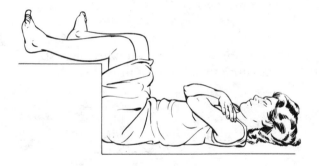

Knee-chest   Chest and side of face down on table, buttocks elevated, knees completely flexed with top of feet on table.

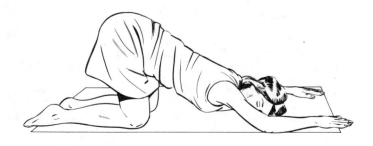

Fowler   Head up, knees at 45° angle, legs down.

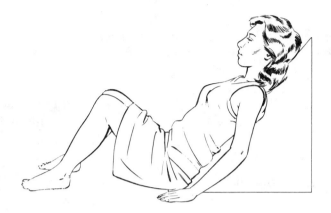

Prone   Face down, opposite of dorsal or supine.

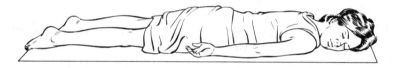

Sims   Lying on left side, knees bent toward abdomen.

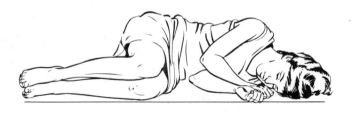

Lateral   Lying on either side, with body at edge of table, lower leg slightly flexed (depending on side lying on), upper leg straight if a pillow is placed between legs, or fully flexed for comfort and ease of examination, arms outstretched at right angles for support.

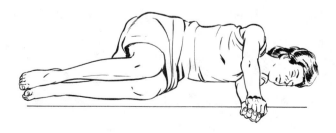

1. POSITIONS AND LOCATIONS MATCHING EXERCISE

Match the following positions and locations in the left column with their definitions in the right column.

_____	1. dorsal	a.	lying on face
_____	2. supine	b.	pertaining to back of body
_____	3. anterior	c.	pertaining to front of body
_____	4. peripheral	d.	inside
_____	5. distal	e.	toward the head
_____	6. external	f.	pertaining to head or skull
_____	7. medial	g.	pertaining to back of body
_____	8. posterior	h.	above
_____	9. cavity	i.	nearest attachment point
_____	10. cranial	j.	near the surface
_____	11. superior	k.	lying on back
_____	12. lateral	l.	farthest from point of attachment
_____	13. prone	m.	pertaining to structures found inside the body
_____	14. ventral	n.	pertaining to front of body
_____	15. visceral	o.	pertaining to lower part of spinal column
_____	16. inferior	p.	toward the midline
_____	17. cephalad	q.	below
_____	18. caudal	r.	pertaining to structure wall
_____	19. proximal	s.	any hollow space
_____	20. internal	t.	outside
_____	21. parietal	u.	pertaining to side of body

2. PREFIX DEFINITION EXERCISE

Underline the prefix in each word and define the prefix in the space provided.

1. intravenous _____

2. retrosternal _____

3. periotic _____

4. ectoderm _____

5. excise _____

6. supralumbar _____

7. antenatal _____

8. prenatal _____

9. postmortem _____

10. neoplasm _____

11. abnormal _____

12. anesthesia _____

13. dehydrate _____

14. hemiplegia _____

15. hypotension _____

16. hypertension _____

17. triangle _____

18. bradycardia _____

19. multicellular _____

20. semiconscious _____

21. tachycardia _____

22. bicuspid _____

23. polyuria _____

24. leucocyte (leukocyte) _____

25. cyanosis _____

26. albumin _____

27. erythrocyte _____

28. ambidextrous _____

29. anteriolateral _____

30. posteriomedial _____

31. dextromanual _____

32. levotorsion _____

33. lateroversion _____

34. mediotarsal _____

35. hydrocephalus _____

36. malnutrition _____

37. biology _____

38. etiology _____

39. narcotic _____

40. micrometer _____

41. megacolon _____

42. panacea _____

43. pyogenic _____

44. febrile _____

45. aerobic _____

46. dysuria _____

47. noctambulism _____

Define the following words.

48. cavity _____

49. proximal _____

50. medial _____

3. MORE PREFIXES DEFINITION EXERCISE

Underline the prefix and define it.

1. periotic _____

2. triangle _____

3. prenatal _____

4.   postnatal _____

5.   anesthesia _____

6.   excise _____

7.   dehydrate _____

8.   hemiplegia _____

9.   intravenous _____

10. bradycardia _____

11. hypoglycemia _____

12. hypertension _____

13. multicellular _____

14. semiconscious _____

15. tachycardia _____

16. bicuspid _____

17. retrosternal _____

18. polyuria _____

19. leucocyte _____

20. cyanosis _____

21. albumin _____

22. erythrocyte _____

23. ambidextrous _____

24. anteriolateral _____

25. posteriomedial _____

26. retrolingual _____

27. supralumbar _____

28. levorotation _____

29. mesoderm _____

30. melanoma _____

31. opisthotic _____

32. diameter _____

33. narcotic _____

34. panacea _____

35. pyogenic _____

36. febrile _____

37. afebrile _____

38. antenatal _____

39. dysuria _____

40. ectoderm _____

Define the following terms.

41. Posterior _____

42. Inferior _____

43. Visceral _____

44. Peripheral _____

45. Prone _____

46. External _____

47. Internal _____

48. Parietal _____

49. Caudal _____

50. Cranial _____

4. PREFIX COMPLETION EXERCISE

Fill in the blanks with the correct prefix.

1. A red cell is called an _____cyte.

2. One who can use both hands is considered to be _____ dextrous.

3. Water in the brain is called _____encephalosis.

4. Nutrition that is bad is called _____nutrition.

5. The study of life is _____logy.

6. An abnormally large colon is called a _____colon.

7. Walking at night (in your sleep) is called _____ambulism.

8. Something causing pus is a _____genic.

9. Something removing fever is called a _____pyrogen.

10. Painful or difficult urination is _____uria.

11. _____dermal means below the skin.

12. Behind the tongue is _____lingual.

13. Before birth is _____natal.

14. After birth is _____natal.

15. To remove water is _____hydrate.

16. A slow heartbeat is _____cardia.

17. A fast heartbeat is _____cardia.

18. _____neural means one nerve.

19. Many cells is _____cellular.

20. A white cell is a _____cyte.

21. Periotic means _____the eye.

22. Upon the skin is _____ dermic.

23. A condition of being blue is _____tic.

24. Something four-footed is called a _____ped.

25. Someone who is thin-skinned could be called _____ dermic.

26. Someone who is abnormally afraid of death is _____ phobic.

27. A condition of having a hidden (or undescended) testicle is _____orchidism.

28. Behind the ear is _____otic.

29. A cure-all is a _____acea.

30. One causing a person to have straight teeth is called an _____dontist.

5. PREFIX PUZZLE

ACROSS

2. Difficult, painful
4. White
8. Slow
9. Against
11. Too little, under, low
15. Middle
17. Many, much
19. Red
22. Before
24. Death
26. He, she, or ———
27. Upon
28. Behind
29. Cause
30. Water
31. Behind
33. Thin
35. ——— off a branch
36. In front
38. Inner, inside
39. Four
40. Pus
43. White
45. Within
48. Night
49. Donkey
51. Put it ———
52. Large
54. Above
55. Fever
57. Both

DOWN

1. Half
3. Under
5. Blue
6. Fast
7. Sweet, sugar
10. New
12. Straight
13. Woman
14. Around
16. On the outside
17. After
18. Sleep
20. Behind
21. Too much, over, high
23. Right
24. Night
25. Hidden
30. Nickname for "honey"
32. Four
34. Fever, fire
35. To the side of
37. Bad
40. All
41. Owns
42. Between
44. Left
46. Before
47. Small
49. From, away
50. Above
52. Very large
53. Away
56. Life
58. In the middle

5. PREFIX PUZZLE

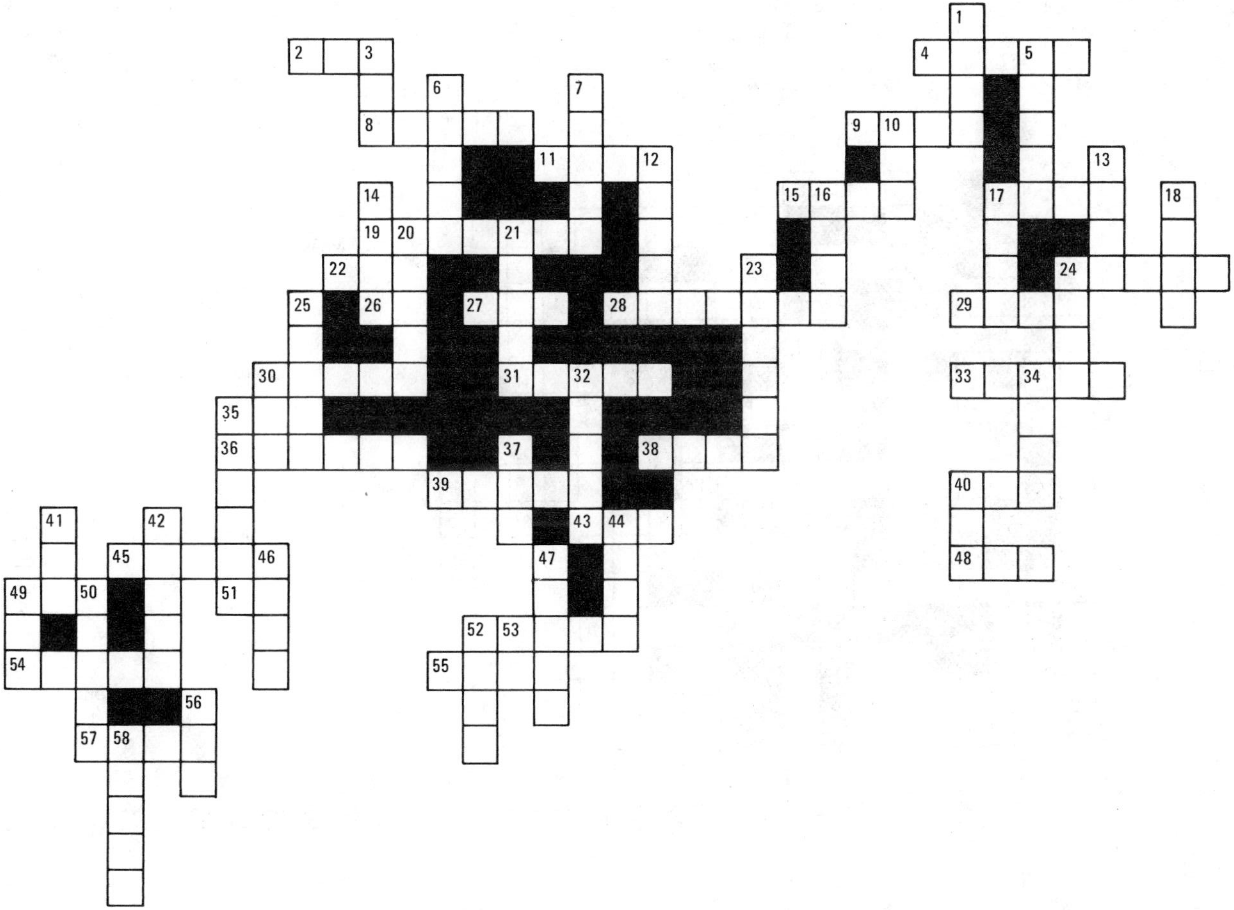

6. MORE PREFIXES, POSITIONS, AND LOCATIONS PUZZLE

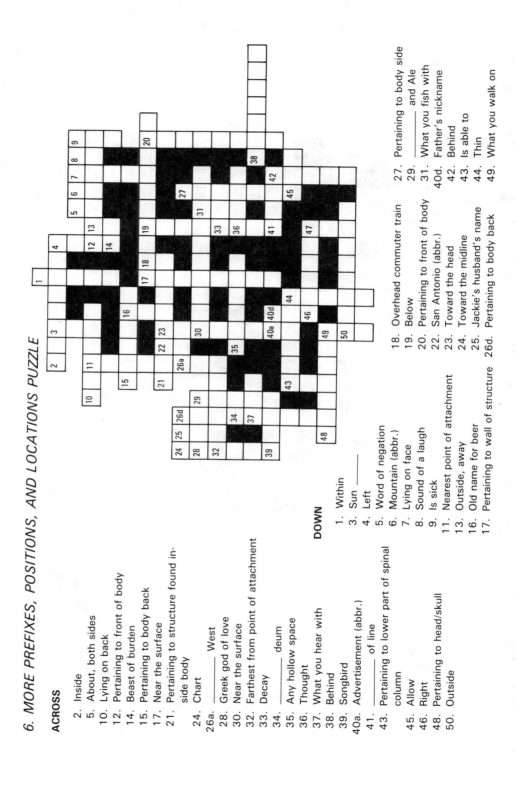

ACROSS

2. Inside
5. About, both sides
10. Lying on back
12. Pertaining to front of body
14. Beast of burden
15. Pertaining to body back
17. Near the surface
21. Pertaining to structure found in-side body
24. Chart
26a. _____ West
28. Greek god of love
30. Near the surface
32. Farthest from point of attachment
33. Decay
34. _____ deum
35. Any hollow space
36. Thought
37. What you hear with
38. Behind
39. Songbird
40a. Advertisement (abbr.)
41. _____ of line
43. Pertaining to lower part of spinal column
45. Allow
46. Right
48. Pertaining to head/skull
50. Outside

DOWN

1. Within
3. Sun _____
4. Left
5. Word of negation
6. Mountain (abbr.)
7. Lying on face
8. Sound of a laugh
9. Is sick
11. Nearest point of attachment
13. Outside, away
16. Old name for beer
17. Pertaining to wall of structure
18. Overhead commuter train
19. Below
20. Pertaining to front of body
22. San Antonio (abbr.)
23. Toward the head
24. Toward the midline
25. Jackie's husband's name
26d. Pertaining to body back
27. Pertaining to body side
29. _____ and Ale
31. What you fish with
40d. Father's nickname
42. Behind
43. Is able to
44. Thin
49. What you walk on

70

7. INCISIONS AND REGIONS PUZZLE

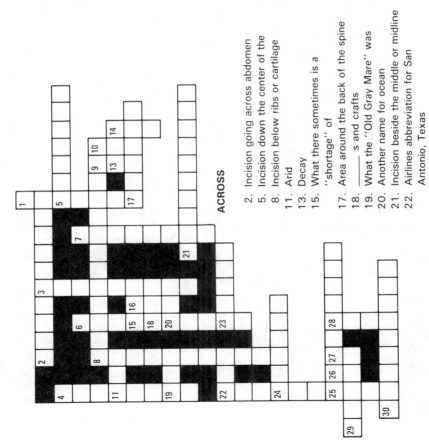

ACROSS

2. Incision going across abdomen
5. Incision down the center of the
8. Incision below ribs or cartilage
11. Arid
13. Decay
15. What there sometimes is a "shortage" of
17. Area around the back of the spine
18. ___ s and crafts
19. What the "Old Gray Mare" was
20. Another name for ocean
21. Incision beside the middle or midline
22. Airlines abbreviation for San Antonio, Texas
23. Incision around the groin or ilium
24. Incision in abdominal muscle
25. Area around "belly button"
29. Area over bone below "belly button"
30. Standard appendectomy incision

DOWN

1. Area in upper thigh, named after bone and artery
3. Area below rib
4. What the abdomen is divided into four of
6. Means upon, over, or beside stomach
7. Area in the groin
8. Area below the stomach
9. What you have two of, that has fingers and hands
10. What an empty ear of corn is called
14. A kind of dance
16. "You ___ there!"
22. Area immediately above bone below belly button
26. Note after "re"
27. Abbreviation for Before Christ
28. What you do when you are against a wall and resting

71

8. ABDOMINAL REGIONS AND INCISIONS PUZZLE

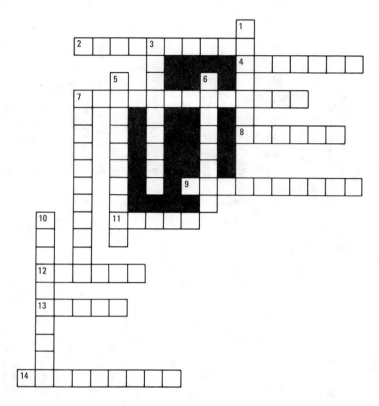

ACROSS

2. Across and above belly button
4. Middle
7. Upper right or left
8. Right or left middle sides

9. Up and down middle
11. Bottom right or left
12. To right of belly button, middle and lower quadrant
13. Above pubic bone, right at it
14. Appendectomy incision

DOWN

1. Right or left thigh
3. Angle across right to middle upper quadrant

5. Middle upper quadrant
6. Right or left lower quadrant
7. Middle lower quadrant
10. Over pubic bone

9. PREFIX MULTIPLE CHOICE EXERCISE

Select the correct answer(s) and write the letter(s) of your choice in the space provided.

_____ 1. A prefix is always found at the
    (a) end of each word.
    (b) middle of each word.
    (c) beginning of each word.
    (d) the beginning or end of each word.

_____ 2. Super means
    (a) great.
    (b) above.
    (c) below.
    (d) between.

_____ 3. Semi means
    (a) about half.
    (b) at least half.
    (c) over half.
    (d) how you cook a steak.

_____ 4. The word for within, or inside, is
    (a) erythro.
    (b) endo.
    (c) external.
    (d) none of the above.

_____ 5. The word for outside is
   (a) extra.
   (b) poly.
   (c) ecto.
   (d) antero.

_____ 6. Dextro means
   (a) sugar.
   (b) left.
   (c) right.
   (d) both.

_____ 7. Ad means
   (a) something selling goods.
   (b) white.
   (c) height.
   (d) near, toward.

_____ 8. The word for above is
   (a) para.
   (b) sub.
   (c) supra.
   (d) super.

_____ 9. Melan means
   (a) watermelon.
   (b) orange.
   (c) black.
   (d) green.

_____ 10. The word for upon is
   (a) epi.
   (b) erythro.
   (c) lipo.
   (d) prone.

_____ 11. Sub means
   (a) across.
   (b) under.
   (c) behind.
   (d) thin.

_____ 12. Necro means
(a) black.
(b) without.
(c) different.
(d) death.

_____ 13. Andro means
(a) man.
(b) woman.
(c) human.
(d) none of the above.

_____ 14. The word for air is
(a) acro.
(b) aero.
(c) ambi.
(d) alb.

_____ 15. Dys means
(a) two, double.
(b) brown.
(c) difficult or painful.
(d) simple.

_____ 16. Latero means
(a) on the left side.
(b) to the side of.
(c) at the bottom of.
(d) rungs on a ladder.

_____ 17. Etio means
(a) cause.
(b) fever.
(c) around.
(d) outside of.

_____ 18. Mono means
(a) kissing disease.
(b) many.
(c) one, single.
(d) more than two.

_____ 19. Para means
(a) above.
(b) beside, near, beyond, or apart from.
(c) around.
(d) after.

_____ 20. A word for white is
(a) alb.
(b) chro.
(c) aero.
(d) ad.

_____ 21. Hypo means
(a) above.
(b) beside.
(c) low.
(d) half.

_____ 22. Neo means
(a) old.
(b) three.
(c) after.
(d) new.

_____ 23. Uni means
(a) items.
(b) one.
(c) too much.
(d) many.

_____ 24. Antero means
(a) in front.
(b) to the side of.
(c) behind.
(d) across.

_____ 25. The word for life is
(a) necro.
(b) bio.
(c) neo.
(d) auto.

_____ 26. Multi means
      (a) too much.
      (b) fast.
      (c) four.
      (d) many.

_____ 27. Anti means
      (a) for.
      (b) against.
      (c) four.
      (d) before.

_____ 28. Ex means
      (a) cause.
      (b) upon.
      (c) past.
      (d) outside, away.

_____ 29. Meso means
      (a) middle.
      (b) top.
      (c) bottom.
      (d) none of the above.

_____ 30. Ab means
      (a) white.
      (b) near to, toward.
      (c) from or away.
      (d) large.

_____ 31. The word for two, or double, is
      (a) bio.
      (b) bi.
      (c) tri.
      (d) multi.

_____ 32. An means
      (a) near to, toward.
      (b) before.
      (c) from, away.
      (d) without.

_____ 33. Tetra means
   (a) snake.
   (b) four.
   (c) three.
   (d) many.

_____ 34. Pyo means
   (a) pus.
   (b) fever.
   (c) around.
   (d) much.

_____ 35. Retro means
   (a) before.
   (b) thin.
   (c) behind.
   (d) small.

_____ 36. Tachy means
   (a) improperly dressed.
   (b) fast.
   (c) slow.
   (d) normal speed.

_____ 37. Peri means
   (a) beside.
   (b) around.
   (c) many, much.
   (d) behind.

_____ 38. Ambi means
   (a) against.
   (b) white.
   (c) about, both sides.
   (d) both.

_____ 39. Micro means
   (a) large.
   (b) very large.
   (c) thin.
   (d) small.

_____   40. Di means
       (a) double or across.
       (b) triple.
       (c) many, much.
       (d) slow.

_____   41. Cyano means
       (a) nose.
       (b) blue.
       (c) black.
       (d) yellow.

_____   42. Opistho means
       (a) eye.
       (b) backward.
       (c) across.
       (d) straight.

_____   43. Medio means
       (a) middle.
       (b) bad.
       (c) black.
       (d) behind.

_____   44. Abs means
       (a) near to, toward.
       (b) white.
       (c) from, away.
       (d) before.

_____   45. Lute means
       (a) an instrument.
       (b) white.
       (c) green.
       (d) yellow.

_____   46. Tele means
       (a) call.
       (b) far-away.
       (c) describe.
       (d) across.

_____ 47. Chro means
  (a) a bird.
  (b) frozen.
  (c) color.
  (d) blue.

_____ 48. Inter means
  (a) between.
  (b) one.
  (c) come inside.
  (d) mix.

_____ 49. Quad means
  (a) three.
  (b) four.
  (c) six.
  (d) shoe width.

_____ 50. The word for behind, or located behind, is
  (a) retro.
  (b) meso.
  (c) endo.
  (d) supra.

_____ 51. Hemi means
  (a) blood.
  (b) double.
  (c) half.
  (d) too much.

_____ 52. Poly means
  (a) parrot.
  (b) many, much.
  (c) about half.
  (d) slow.

_____ 53. Lepto means
  (a) butterfly.
  (b) fat.
  (c) large.
  (d) thin.

_____ 54. Ortho means
   (a) straight.
   (b) teeth.
   (c) bone.
   (d) behind.

_____ 55. Pan means
   (a) all.
   (b) bread.
   (c) sides.
   (d) sugar.

_____ 56. Hetero means
   (a) uterus.
   (b) too much.
   (c) same.
   (d) different.

_____ 57. Noct means
   (a) middle.
   (b) night.
   (c) rap.
   (d) sleep.

_____ 58. Febr means
   (a) pus.
   (b) woman.
   (c) fever.
   (d) sweet.

_____ 59. Hyper means
   (a) not enough.
   (b) slow.
   (c) too much.
   (d) fast.

_____ 60. Brady means
   (a) slow.
   (b) fast.
   (c) under.
   (d) across.

_____ 61. Trans means
    (a) four.
    (b) green.
    (c) far away.
    (d) across.

_____ 62. Leuco means
    (a) blood disease.
    (b) white.
    (c) yellow.
    (d) middle.

_____ 63. Erythro means
    (a) outside of.
    (b) cause.
    (c) red.
    (d) four.

_____ 64. De means
    (a) remove, from.
    (b) two, double.
    (c) difficult, painful.
    (d) too much.

_____ 65. Mega means
    (a) abnormally small.
    (b) abnormally large.
    (c) abnormally short.
    (d) abnormally tall.

_____ 66. Gyne means
    (a) behind.
    (b) man.
    (c) woman.
    (d) sugar.

_____ 67. Gluc means
    (a) woman.
    (b) around.
    (c) sweet, sugar.
    (d) half.

_____ 68. Pre means

    (a) new.

    (b) after.

    (c) under.

    (d) before.

_____ 69. Post means

    (a) before.

    (b) after.

    (c) beside.

    (d) behind.

_____ 70. Narc means

    (a) drug.

    (b) night.

    (c) sleep.

    (d) death.

_____ 71. Mal means

    (a) bad.

    (b) good.

    (c) indifferent.

    (d) black.

_____ 72. Amphi means

    (a) air.

    (b) without.

    (c) near to.

    (d) both sides.

_____ 73. Crypt means

    (a) grave.

    (b) hidden.

    (c) beneath.

    (d) death.

_____ 74. Acro means

    (a) height.

    (b) large.

    (c) both.

    (d) near to.

_____ 75. Gyne means
    (a) sweet, sugar.
    (b) woman.
    (c) slow.
    (d) hysterical.

_____ 76. Hydro means
    (a) half.
    (b) too much.
    (c) water.
    (d) different.

_____ 77. Levo means
    (a) thin.
    (b) white.
    (c) to the side of.
    (d) left.

_____ 78. Postero means
    (a) behind.
    (b) fever, fire.
    (c) backward.
    (d) beside, near.

_____ 79. Pyro means
    (a) fever, fire.
    (b) pus.
    (c) disease.
    (d) near.

_____ 80. Lipo means
    (a) stone.
    (b) left.
    (c) fat.
    (d) thin.

ZEROING IN ON
SUFFIXES

4

A suffix is a syllable or combination of letters found at the end of a word which adds to the meaning of the word. Note: Several syllables used here as suffixes are also used as root or stem words.

SUFFIXES

Suffix	Meaning	Word Example
algia	pain	neuralgia
archy	rule	anarchy
cele	swelling, hernia, protrusion	hydrocele
centesis	puncture of and withdrawal of fluid	amniocentesis
cide	kill	homicide
cise	cut	excise
cle	small	cuticle, corpuscle
cule	small	molecule
cyte	cell	leucocyte
duct	to lead	oviduct, abduct
dyne, dynia	pain	anodyne, cardiodynia

SUFFIXES

Suffix	Meaning	Word Example
ecta, ectasis	extension, dilations	ureterectasis
ectomy	surgical removal	appendectomy
ectop, ectopy	displacement, mal-position, especially congenital (*ec*, out of; *topy*, place)	splenectopy
ele, elle	small	organelle
emesis	vomiting	hematemesis
emia	condition of the blood	anemia, hypo-glycemia
ens	of, belonging to	(homo) sapiens
esthesia	sensation, feeling	anesthesia
eum	a place where	museum
form	resembling, shaped	fusiform
ful	full of	wonderful
gen	produce	antigen
genic	produced by, producing	pyogenic, pathogenic
gram	instrument that records lines or drawings	cardiogram
graph	lines, drawings, writing	cardiograph
iasis	process, condition, presence of	lithiasis
icle	little	testicle, icicle, popsicle
id	condition of	morbid, rabid
ion	small	clarion, solion
ist	one who	cardiologist
itis	inflammation of, infection	endocarditis, hepatitis
ium	small	pericardium
ize	away, remove, free from	cauterize

SUFFIXES

Suffix	Meaning	Word Example
lepsy	seizure	narcolepsy
lith	stone	cholelithiasis
logy	study of, science	biology
lysis	destruction, decomposition, dissolution	paralysis
lytic	gradual abatement or lessening of the symptoms of disease	biolytic
megaly	enlargement	cardiomegaly
malacia	morbid softening	osteomalacia
metry	measurement	telemetry
mit	sent, full of	transmit
oda, odes	like, a resemblance	electrodes
oid	resembling, form	ovoid, android, rheumatoid
ola, ole	small	arteriola, vacuole
ology	study of, science	histology
oma	growth, tumor	hepatoma
os	opening or mouth	ileostomy
osis	process, condition of, disease	diagnosis
ostomy	opening formed for drainage	colostomy, tracheostomy
otomy	incision	tracheotomy
ous	full of, having	subcutaneous
parous	giving birth to, bearing	multiparous
pathy	disease	neuropathy
ped, pedi	foot, child	orthopedics
pedia	education	encyclopedia
pedia	child	pediatrician
penia	too few	leukocytopenia
pexy	surgical fixation	hysteropexy

SUFFIXES

Suffix	Meaning	Word Example
phag, phago	swallowing, eating	aphagia, phago-cytosis, esophagus
phasia	speech	aphasia
phobia	abnormal fear, dread	photophobia, hydrophobia
phyll	leaf	chlorophyll
plasm	anything formed	ectoplasm
plast	anything formed	neoplast
plasty	repair, molding	rhinoplasty
pnea	breathing	apnea; dyspnea
pod	foot	pseudopod
ptosis	dropping of an organ	proctoptosis
ptysis	spitting, saliva	hemoptysis
rrhage	bursting forth	hemorrhage
rrhea	flow	diarrhea, dysmenorrhea
rrhaphy	suture, repair	herniorrhaphy
rrhexis	break, rupture	cardiorrhexis
sclere, sclero	hard	arteriosclerosis
scope	instrument to examine	microscope, telescope
scopy	examine, observation	endoscopy
sis	act of	uresis
sophy	wisdom, art, skill	philosophy
spasm	involuntary muscular act; convulsion; twitching	neurospasm
spire	breath	respiration
stalsis	constriction, compression	peristalsis
stom, stoma	opening into; a mouth; artificial opening	astomia
taxis	arrangement	taxidermist

SUFFIXES

Suffix	Meaning	Word Example
tax, taxo	arrangement	taxonomy
tic	belonging to	periotic
tomy	cutting, incision	myringotomy, laparotomy
trophy	nourishment	atrophy, dystrophy
tropic	turning toward; tending to turn or change	inotropic
tropism	growth response stimulus	phototropism
ule	small	granule
ulum, ulus	small	ovulum, homunculus
uria	in the urine	hematuria

DIAGNOSTIC AND SYMPTOMATIC TERMS

Suffix	Meaning
algia	pain
cele	swelling, hernia
ecta, ectasis	extension, dilation
emia	condition of the blood
genic	caused by
lysis	destruction or decomposition, dissolution; the gradual abatement or receding of the symptoms of disease
malacia	morbid softening of part or morbid craving for highly spiced foods
megaly	enlargement
oid	resembling
oma	growth, tumor
osis	condition of, process, disease
pathy	disease
penia	too few
ptosis	dropping of an organ

DIAGNOSTIC AND SYMPTOMATIC TERMS

Suffix	Meaning
ptysis	spitting or saliva
rrhagia	bursting forth
rrhea	flow
rrhexis	break, rupture
sclere, sclero	hard
spasm	involuntary muscular act; convulsion
trophy	nourishment

OPERATIVE OR SURGICAL FIELD

Suffix	Meaning
centesis	puncture of and withdrawal of fluid
desis	binding
ectomy	surgical removal of
ostomy	opening, mouthlike (os)
otomy	incision
pexy	surgical fixation
plasty	repair, molding
rrhaphy	suture, repair
scopy	to examine or observe

1. SUFFIX DEFINITION EXERCISE

In this exercise, you are given a medical term. The prefix is defined for you; define the suffix and whole word in the blank.

1. Neur = nerve. Neuralgia = _____ .

2. An = without, or lack. Anarchy = _____ .

3. Hydro = water. Hydrocele = _____ .

4. Amnio = the fluid in amniotic sac surrounding fetus. Amnio-

    centesis = _____ .

5. Patri = father. Patricide = _____ .

6. Ex = away from, or remove. Excise = _____ .

7. Cuti = outer layer or skin. Cuticle = _____ .

8. Ovi = ovum, or egg. Oviduct = _____ .

9. Ab = absence, away from, a term of negation. Abduct =

    _____ .

10. Cardio = heart. Cardiodynia = _____ .

11. Oophor = ovary. Oophorectomy = _____ .

12. Hemat = blood. Hematemesis = _____ .

13. Hypo = below; glyc = sugar. Hypoglycemia = _____ .

14. An = lack of. Anesthesia = _____ .

15. Patho = germs, bacteria. Pathogenic = _____ .

16. Pyo = pus. Pyogenic = _____ .

17. Cardio = pertaining to the heart. Cardiograph = _____

    _____ .

18. Lith = stone. Lithiasis = _____ .

19. Test(i), = the testis, or male gonad. Testicle literally translates

    to _____ .

20. Endo = within; card = heart. Endocarditis = _____ .

21. Peri = around; card = heart. Pericardium = _____ .

22. Narc(o) = sleep. Narcolepsy = _____ .

23. Chole = the bladder (specifically, gall bladder);

lith = stone. Cholelithiasis = _____ .

24. Bio = life. Biology = _____ .

25. Do this one by yourself: cardiomegaly = _____ .

26. Tele = (far) away. Telemetry = _____ .

27. Trans = across. Transmit = _____ .

28. Andr(o) is man. Android = _____ .

29. Histo = tissue. Histology = _____ .

30. Hepat = liver. Hepatoma = _____ .

31. Trache(o) = trachea, or windpipe. Tracheostomy = _____

_____ .

32. Multi = many. Multiparous = _____ .

33. Neuro = nerve. Neuropathy = _____ .

34. Ortho = straight. Literally, orthopedics = _____ .

35. Leuko = white; cyto = cells. Leukocytopenia = _____

_____ .

36. Another one to figure out: phagocytosis = _____

_____ .

37. Mast = breast. Mastopexy = _____ .

38. A = without. Aphasia = _____ .

39. Photo = light. Photophobia = _____ .

40. Hydro = water. Hydrophobia = _____ .

41. Chloro = green. Chlorophyll = _____ .

42. Neo = new. Neoplasm = _____ .

43. Rhino = nose. Rhinoplasty = _____ .

44. Dys = difficult or painful. Dyspnea = _____ .

45. Pseudo = false. Pseudopod = _____ .

46. Procto = rectum or anus. Proctoptosis = _____

_____ .

47. Hemo = blood. Hemoptysis = _____ .

48. Hemorrhage = _____ .

49. Dys = difficult or painful; meno = menstruation. Dysme-

norrhea _____ .

50. Herni(o) = hernia, or rupture. Herniorrhaphy = _____

_____ .

51. Arterior = artery. Arteriosclerosis = _____

_____ . (Look carefully—scler and osis

are both in this word).

52. Micro refers to something small. Microscope = _____

_____ .

53. Endo = within. Endoscopy = _____ .

54. Ure = urine. Uresis = _____ .

54. Ex = form of negation, or lack of. Expiration = _____

   _____ .

55. Peri = around. Peristalsis = _____ .

56. Col(o) = colon. Colostomy = _____ .

57. Taxi(s) = arrangement; derm = skin. Taxidermist = _____

   _____ .

58. Lapar(o) = abdomen. Laparotomy = _____ .

59. Atrophy = _____ .

60. Ino = within. Inotropic = _____ .

61. Hematuria = _____ .

62. Lymph = water. Lymphoma = _____ .

63. Append = the appendix, or something hanging on. Appendectomy = _____ .

64. Psycho = mind. Psychogenic = _____ .

65. Psychosis = _____ .

66. Septic = bacteria. Septicemia = _____ .

67. Pneumo = lung. Pneumocentesis = _____ .

68. Hepato = liver. Hepatomegaly = _____ .

69. Masto = breast. Mastoplasty = _____ .

70. Nost = return home. Nostalgia = _____ .

2. SUFFIX MATCHING EXERCISE

Match the definition in the left column with the suffix in the right column.

_____	1.	abnormal fear of, dread	a. taxis
_____	2.	act of	b. stalsis
_____	3.	anything formed	c. pedia
_____	4.	arrangement	d. phobia
_____	5.	away, remove, free from	e. id
_____	6.	breath, breathing	f. tomy
_____	7.	breathing, breath	g. scopy
_____	8.	bursting forth	h. cise
_____	9.	condition of	i. plast
_____	10.	condition of	j. pathy
_____	11.	condition of the blood	k. ful
_____	12.	constriction, compression	l. ptosis
_____	13.	cut	m. ped
_____	14.	cutting, incision	n. spire
_____	15.	destruction, decomposition	o. rrhea
_____	16.	disease	p. osis
_____	17.	displacement, malposition	q. rrhage
_____	18.	dropping of an organ	r. pod
_____	19.	education, child	s. lysis
_____	20.	enlargement	t. sis
_____	21.	examine, observation	u. emia
_____	22.	flow	v. pnea
_____	23.	foot	w. ectopy
_____	24.	foot, child	x. megaly
_____	25.	full of	y. ize

3. SUFFIX MATCHING EXERCISE

Match the definition in the left column with the suffix in the right column.

_____	1. giving birth to	a.	graph
_____	2. hard	b.	archy
_____	3. in the urine	c.	scope
_____	4. incision	d.	gram
_____	5. inflammation, infection	e.	trophy
_____	6. instrument to examine	f.	cise
_____	7. kill	g.	algia
_____	8. like, resemblance	h.	parous
_____	9. lines, drawings, writing	i.	oid
_____	10. measurement	j.	uria
_____	11. nourishment	k.	ens
_____	12. of, belonging to	l.	lepsy
_____	13. opening, mouth	m.	dyne
_____	14. opening	n.	itis
_____	15. opening into, communication between	o.	osis
_____	16. pain	p.	cide
_____	17. pain	q.	ostomy
_____	18. process, condition of, disease	r.	centesis
_____	19. produced by, producing	s.	metry
_____	20. puncture of and withdrawal of fluid	t.	plasty
_____	21. record	u.	odes
_____	22. repair, molding	v.	os
_____	23. resembling, form	w.	stomy
_____	24. rule	x.	genic
_____	25. seizure	y.	sclero

4. SUFFIX MATCHING EXERCISE

Match the definition in the left column with the suffix in the right column.

_____	1.	sensation, feeling	a.	cule
_____	2.	sent, full of	b.	phasy
_____	3.	small	c.	cele
_____	4.	small	d.	sophy
_____	5.	small	e.	ology
_____	6.	small	f.	esthesia
_____	7.	small	g.	ule
_____	8.	speech	h.	penia
_____	9.	speech	i.	lith
_____	10.	spitting, saliva	j.	elle
_____	11.	stone	k.	ptysis
_____	12.	study of, science	l.	emesis
_____	13.	study of, science	m.	rrhaphy
_____	14.	surgical removal	n.	phasia
_____	15.	suture, repair	o.	duct
_____	16.	swallowing, eating	p.	mit
_____	17.	swelling, hernia	q.	logy
_____	18.	to lead	r.	ole
_____	19.	too few	s.	tropic
_____	20.	tumor, growth	t.	ectomy
_____	21.	turning toward, tending to turn/change	u.	cle
_____	22.	vomiting	v.	oma
_____	23.	wisdom, art, skill	w.	phag

5. SUFFIX MATCHING EXERCISE

In the space provided, match the correct word in the right column with its suffix meaning (in italic) in the left column.

_____	1. new growth, tumor	a. rheumat*oid*
_____	2. inflammation	b. arterio*sclerosis*
_____	3. in the urine	c. append*ectomy*
_____	4. process, condition	d. nephr*optosis*
_____	5. resembling	e. homi*cide*
_____	6. disease	f. hepat*oma*
_____	7. producing, produced by	g. hemo*lysis*
_____	8. vomiting	h. eso*phagus*
_____	9. too few	i. broncho*scopy*
_____	10. swallowing	j. hepat*itis*
_____	11. repair	k. an*esthesia*
_____	12. breathing	l. dys*pnea*
_____	13. dropping of an organ	m. hemat*uria*
_____	14. spitting, saliva	n. cysto*cele*
_____	15. bursting forth	o. leukocyto*penia*
_____	16. flow	p. steri*lize*
_____	17. fear of	q. colo*stomy*
_____	18. suture, repair	r. adeno*pathy*
_____	19. hard	s. hydro*phobia*
_____	20. examination	t. ano*dyne*
_____	21. opening	u. arterioscler*osis*
_____	22. incision	v. hemat*emesis*
_____	23. pain	w. hemo*rrhage*
_____	24. swelling, hernia	x. tracheo*tomy*
_____	25. kill	y. an*emia*
_____	26. cut	z. epi*lepsy*
_____	27. pain	aa. patho*genic*
_____	28. surgical removal	bb. rhino*plasty*
_____	29. blood	cc. hemo*ptysis*

_____	30.	sensation, feeling
_____	31.	record
_____	32.	lines or drawings
_____	33.	away, remove
_____	34.	seizure
_____	35.	study of, science
_____	36.	receding of disease symptoms

dd. hernio*rrhaphy*
ee. neur*algia*
ff. cardio*gram*
gg. psycho*logy*
hh. dia*rrhea*
ii. ex*cise*
jj. cardio*graph*

6. SUFFIX PUZZLE

The clues for this puzzle are on the following page.

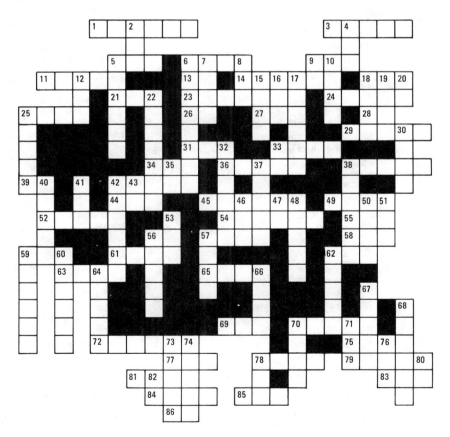

6. SUFFIX PUZZLE

ACROSS

1. Spitting, saliva
3. Examine
5. The Boy King
6. Condition of the blood
9. Small
11. Hard
13. Note after ''fa''
14. Hard
18. Foot
21. What one rows with
23. Turning
24. Produced by, producing
25. Swallowing, eating
26. Masculine pronoun
27. Membership fee
28. Nickname for Edward
29. Process, condition
31. Tree fluid
33. Cut
34. Greek letter
36. Receding of disease symptoms
38. Too few
39. English ''bye''
42. Flow
44. A little _____ of sunshine
45. Opening
49. Cutting, incising
52. Lines or drawings
54. One who taps
55. Honey _____
56. It stinks (abbr.)
57. Pain
58. Small
59. Actress _____ West
61. Record
62. Animal foot
63. Small
65. Swelling, hernia
69. Away, remove, free from
70. Study of, science
72. What makes bread rise
75. Margarine
77. Dined
78. In the urine
79. Anything formed
81. Arrangement
83. Tear
84. What _____ is it?
85. Please eat oranges (abbr.)
86. South Yorkshire (abbr.)

DOWN

2. Pronoun
4. Small
5. Turning
6. Sensation, feeling
7. _____ or less
8. Cleo's snake
9. _____ else
10. Study of, science
12. Dogs have four of these
15. Kill
16. La. State Univ.
17. Vomiting
18. Breathing
19. Resembling
20. Where U.S. capital is
22. Suture, repair
25. Anything formed
30. Inflammation of
32. Repair
33. Coney Island
35. Masculine pronoun
37. Instrument to examine
38. Fear of
40. Pain
41. Growth, tumor
42. Bursting forth
43. Egyptian god
46. Sun _____
47. Military Police
48. Long for
50. Cat's _____
51. Japanese money
53. Small
56. Disease
57. To lead
59. Enlargement
60. Surgical removal
62. Swallowing, eating
64. Seizure
66. Small
67. Leaf
68. Dropping of an organ
70. Process, condition
71. Republican Party
73. Arrangement
74. Opening
76. Hearing organ
78. Small
80. Member of Parliament
82. Location

7. SUFFIX MULTIPLE CHOICE EXERCISE

Select the correct answer(s) and write the letter(s) of your choice in the space provided.

_____   1.   The suffix for constriction is
   (a) emesis.
   (b) iasis.
   (c) rrhexis.
   (d) stalsis.

_____   2.   The suffix for flow is
   (a) rrhage.
   (b) emesis.
   (c) plast.
   (d) rrhea.

_____   3.   The suffix for turning toward is
   (a) tropic.
   (b) taxis.
   (c) spire.
   (d) parous.

_____   4.   The suffix for study of, or science, is
   (a) logy.
   (b) lysis.
   (c) lepsy.
   (d) lytic.

_____   5.   The suffix for suture or repair is
   (a) rrhaphy.
   (b) rrhage.
   (c) rrhea.
   (d) rrhexis.

_____   6. The suffix for nourishment is
          (a) phobia.
          (b) phasia.
          (c) trophy.
          (d) phago.

_____   7. The suffix for in the urine is
          (a) osis.
          (b) uria.
          (c) itis.
          (d) ule.

_____   8. The suffix for disease is
          (a) osis.
          (b) itis.
          (c) pathy.
          (d) plasty.

_____   9. The suffix for incision is
          (a) ostomy.
          (b) cise.
          (c) oda.
          (d) otomy.

_____   10. The suffix for opening is
          (a) cele.
          (b) pexy.
          (c) ostomy.
          (d) otomy.

_____   11. The suffix for process, condition of, or disease is
          (a) ectasis
          (b) osis.
          (c) ectomy.
          (d) emesis.

_____   12. The suffix for growth or tumor is
          (a) pathy.
          (b) lysis.
          (c) oma.
          (d) itis.

_____ 13. The suffix for enlargement is

    (a) trophy.

    (b) spasm.

    (c) algia.

    (d) megaly.

_____ 14. The suffix for free from or remove is

    (a) eum.

    (b) ize.

    (c) phyll.

    (d) rrhexis.

_____ 15. The suffix for inflammation of is

    (a) itis.

    (b) osis.

    (c) pathy.

    (d) rrhea.

_____ 16. The suffix for condition of is

    (a) itis.

    (b) id.

    (c) ostomy.

    (d) esthesia.

_____ 17. The suffix for record is

    (a) gram.

    (b) graph.

    (c) pathy.

    (d) pedia.

_____ 18. The suffix for produced by is

    (a) uria.

    (b) genic.

    (c) itis.

    (d) osis.

_____ 19. The suffix for to lead is

    (a) lytic.

    (b) spire.

    (c) duct.

    (d) sis.

_____ 20. The suffix for condition of blood is
    (a) rrhage.
    (b) osis.
    (c) iasis.
    (d) emia.

_____ 21. The suffix for lines or drawings is
    (a) graph.
    (b) gram.
    (c) genic.
    (d) gen.

_____ 22. The suffix for breathing is
    (a) pnea.
    (b) spire.
    (c) cide.
    (d) ion.

_____ 23. The suffix for repair or molding is
    (a) lith.
    (b) taxis.
    (c) plasty.
    (d) algia.

_____ 24. The suffix for process, condition, or presence is
    (a) oid.
    (b) itis.
    (c) osis.
    (d) iasis.

_____ 25. The suffix for speech is
    (a) phasia.
    (b) ptosis.
    (c) ptysis.
    (d) pexy.

_____ 26. The suffix for spitting or saliva is
    (a) pnea.
    (b) ptysis.
    (c) ptosis.
    (d) ule.

_____ 27. The suffix for break or rupture is
     (a) rrhea.
     (b) rrhexis.
     (c) rrhage.
     (d) rrhaphy.

_____ 28. The suffix for sensation or feeling is
     (a) ectasis.
     (b) esthesia.
     (c) lysis.
     (d) itis.

_____ 29. The suffix for stone is
     (a) sophy.
     (b) stoma.
     (c) lytic.
     (d) lith.

_____ 30. The suffix for surgical removal is
     (a) ectomy.
     (b) ectopy.
     (c) ectasis.
     (d) elle.

_____ 31. The suffix for surgical fixation is
     (a) rrhaphy.
     (b) pexy.
     (c) tomy.
     (d) taxis.

_____ 32. The suffix for cutting, incision, is
     (a) itis.
     (b) tomy.
     (c) osis.
     (d) ptosis.

_____ 33. The suffix for vomiting is
     (a) itis.
     (b) centesis.
     (c) emesis.
     (d) lepsy.

_____ 34. The suffix for pain is
    (a) duct.
    (b) dyne.
    (c) archy.
    (d) algia.

_____ 35. The suffix for cutting or incision is
    (a) algia.
    (b) otomy.
    (c) centesis.
    (d) uria.

_____ 36. The suffix for instrument to examine is
    (a) metry.
    (b) lytic.
    (c) scope.
    (d) taxis.

_____ 37. The suffix for belonging to is
    (a) archy.
    (b) tic.
    (c) lepsy.
    (d) uria.

_____ 38. The suffix for bursting forth is
    (a) lysis.
    (b) rrhage.
    (c) trophy.
    (d) rrhea.

_____ 39. The suffix for dropping of an organ is
    (a) rrhaphy.
    (b) plasty.
    (c) ptosis.
    (d) ptysis.

_____ 40. The suffix for swallowing or eating is
    (a) osis.
    (b) oma.
    (c) stomy.
    (d) phag.

_____ 41. The suffix for too few is
    (a) pedia.
    (b) pnea.
    (c) penia.
    (d) sophy.

_____ 42. The suffix for swelling or hernia is
    (a) sclero.
    (b) cele.
    (c) pathy.
    (d) icle.

_____ 43. The suffix for abnormal fear or dread is
    (a) phobia.
    (b) algia.
    (c) dyne.
    (d) phasia.

_____ 44. The suffix for destruction is
    (a) centesis.
    (b) itis.
    (c) osis.
    (d) lysis.

_____ 45. The suffix for measurement is
    (a) penia.
    (b) megaly.
    (c) metry.
    (d) ostomy.

_____ 46. The suffix for kill is
    (a) necro.
    (b) cele.
    (c) cide.
    (d) cise.

_____ 47. The suffix for full of is
    (a) ful.
    (b) cle.
    (c) eum.
    (d) osis.

_____ 48. The suffix for opening or mouth is
   (a) itis.
   (b) phyll.
   (c) os.
   (d) ful.

_____ 49. The suffix for produce is
   (a) gen.
   (b) cle.
   (c) parous.
   (d) plasty.

_____ 50. The suffix for cut is
   (a) emia.
   (b) ectopy.
   (c) ectomy.
   (d) cise.

GETTING DOWN TO
ROOTS
5

The root is the main body, or the basic component, of a word.

ROOTS

Root	Meaning	Word Example
aden, adeno	gland	adenopathy
andr, andro	man	android
angi, angio	vessel	angiogram
arthr, arthro	joint	arthritis
bronch, broncho	bronchus	bronchitis
cardi, cardio	heart	endocarditis
cephal, cephalo	head	hydrocephalus
chil, chilo	lip	lipochilo
chol, chole	bile, gall	cholangiogram
chondr, chondro	cartilage	chondroma
cili, cilia, cilio	eyelid, small hair, eyelash	ciliectomy
col, colo	colon	colitis
colp, colpo, colpos	vagina	colporrhaphy
corpus	body	corpuscle

ROOTS

Root	Meaning	Word Example
cost, costo	rib	intercostal
cry, cryo	freeze, cold	cryesthesia
cut, cuti, cutane	skin	cuticle
cyst, cysto	sac, bladder	cystitis
cyt, cyto	cell	cytology
dent, denti, dento	tooth	dentist
derm, derma	skin	dermatitis
enter, entero	intestine	enteritis
fibr, fibro	connective tissue	fibroma
gastr, gastro	stomach	gastroenteritis, gastrectomy
glob, globo	ball, globe	hemoglobin
gloss, glosso	tongue	glossitis
hem, hemo	blood	hemopathy
hemat, hemato	blood	hematocytopenia
hepat, hepato	liver	hepatitis
hist, histo	tissue	histogram
hyster, hystero	uterus	oophoro-hysterectomy
kerat, kerato	horn, cornea	keratosis, keratalgia
lapar, laparo	loins, abdomen	laparotomy
lingu, linguo	tongue	bilingual
lip, lipo	fat	lipoma
lith, litho	stone	cholelithiasis
mast, masto	breast	mastectomy
muc, muco	mucus	mucocele
my, myo	muscle	endomyocarditis
myc, myco	fungus	mycology
nas, naso	nose	nasogastritis
nephr, nephro	renal, kidney	nephrolithiasis
neur, neuro	nerve	neuropathic

ROOTS

Root	Meaning	Word Example
ocul, oculo	eye	oculist
oophor, oophoro	ovary	oophorectomy
ophthalm, ophthalmo	eye	ophthalmologist
optic	eye	optician
oro, ora, ori	an opening, or mouth	oral, orad
orchi, orchio	testicle, testis	cryptorchidism
oste, osteo	bone	osteoarthritis
ot, oti, oto	ear	otitis
otic	ear	otic
ped (Greek)	child	pediatrician
ped (Latin)	foot	orthopedics, biped
phleb, phlebo	vein	phlebitis
pneum, pneumo	lung, air	pneumonitis
proct, procto	rectum, anus	proctoscope
psyche, psycho	mind	psychogenic
pyel, pyelo	kidney pelvis (renal pelvis)	pyelonephritis
renal	pertaining to the kidney	renal
ren, reni	kidney	renopathy
rhin, rhino	nose	rhinitis
salping, salpingo	tube	salpingogram
thorac, thoraco	chest, thorax	pneumothoracic, thoracentesis
thromb, thrombo	clot	thrombophlebitis
tinea	fungus	tinea pedia
vas, vaso	blood vessel, vessel, or duct	vas deferens, vasectomy, vasoconstriction

1. ROOT MATCHING EXERCISE

Match the root in the left column with the correct definition in the right column.

_____	1. aden, adeno	a.	vessel
_____	2. andr, andro	b.	vein
_____	3. angi, angio	c.	vagina
_____	4. arthr, arthro	d.	uterus
_____	5. bronch, broncho	e.	tube
_____	6. cardi, cardio	f.	tooth
_____	7. cephal, cephalo	g.	tongue
_____	8. chil, chilo	h.	tongue
_____	9. chol, chole	i.	tissue
_____	10. chondr, chondro	j.	testicle, testis
_____	11. cili, cilia, cilio	k.	stone
_____	12. col, colo	l.	stomach
_____	13. colp, colpo	m.	skin
_____	14. corpus	n.	skin
_____	15. cost, costo	o.	sac, bladder
_____	16. cryo	p.	rib
_____	17. cut, cuti	q.	renal, kidney
_____	18. cyst, cysto	r.	rectum, anus
_____	19. cyt, cyto	s.	pertaining to kidney
_____	20. dent, denti, dento	t.	kidney (renal) pelvis
_____	21. derm, derma	u.	ovary
_____	22. enter, entero	v.	stomach–mouth opening
_____	23. fibr, fibro	w.	nose
_____	24. gastr, gastro	x.	nose
_____	25. glob, globo	y.	nerve
_____	26. gloss, glosso	z.	muscle
_____	27. hem, hemo	aa.	mucus
_____	28. hemat, hemato	bb.	mouths
_____	29. hepat, hepato	cc.	mouth
_____	30. hist, histo	dd.	mind
_____	31. hyster, hystero	ee.	man
_____	32. kerat, kerato	ff.	lung, air
_____	33. lapar, laparo	gg.	loins, abdomen

_____	34. lingu, linguo	hh.	liver
_____	35. lip, lipo	ii.	lip
_____	36. lith, litho	jj.	joint
_____	37. mast, masto	kk.	intestine
_____	38. muc, muco	ll.	horn, cornea
_____	39. my, myo	mm.	heart
_____	40. myc, myco	nn.	head
_____	41. nas, naso	oo.	gland
_____	42. nephr, nephro	pp.	fungus
_____	43. neur, neuro	qq.	fungus
_____	44. ocul, oculo	rr.	freeze, cold
_____	45. oophor, oophoro	ss.	foot
_____	46. ophthalm	tt.	fat
_____	47. optic	uu.	eyelid/lash, small hair
_____	48. or, oro	vv.	eye
_____	49. ora	ww.	eye
_____	50. orchi, orchio	xx.	eye
_____	51. os	yy.	pertaining to ear
_____	52. oste, osteo	zz.	ear
_____	53. ot, oto, oti	aaa.	connective tissue
_____	54. otic	bbb.	colon
_____	55. ped (Greek)	ccc.	clot
_____	56. ped (Latin)	ddd.	child
_____	57. phleb, phlebo	eee.	chest or thorax
_____	58. pneum, pneumo	fff.	cell
_____	59. proct, procto	ggg.	cartilage
_____	60. psyche, psycho	hhh.	bronchus
_____	61. pyel, pyelo	iii.	breast
_____	62. renal	jjj.	bone
_____	63. rhin, rhino	kkk.	body
_____	64. salping, salpingo	lll.	blood vessel, vessel, duct
_____	65. thorac, thoraco	mmm.	blood vessel, vessel, duct
_____	66. thromb, thrombo	nnn.	blood
_____	67. tinea	ooo.	blood
_____	68. vas	ppp.	bile, gall
_____	69. vas, vaso	qqq.	ball, globe

2. ROOT IDENTIFICATION EXERCISE

Write the proper root for the following words.

1. bile _____

2. blood _____

3. blood (another term) _____

4. body _____

5. cartilage _____

6. cell _____

7. colon _____

8. connective tissue _____

9. fat _____

10. head _____

11. heart _____

12. horn, cornea _____

13. intestine _____

14. joint _____

15. man _____

16. mucus _____

17. rib _____

18. sac, bladder _____

19. skin _____

20. stone _____

21. tissue _____

22. tongue _____

23. tongue (another term) _____

24. tooth _____

25. vagina _____

3. ROOT DEFINITION EXERCISE

Write the proper root for each definition.

1. blood vessel _____

2. bone _____

3. clot _____

4. chest _____

5. child _____

6. ear _____

7. ear (another term) _____

8. eye _____

9. eye (another term) _____

10. foot _____

11. fungus _____

12. kidney, renal _____

13. lung, air _____

14. mind _____

15. mouth _____

16. muscle _____

17. nerve _____

18. nose _____

19. nose (another term) _____

20. opening _____

21. ovary _____

22. pelvis of kidney _____

23. pertaining to the kidney _____

24. tube _____

25. vessel, duct _____

4. ROOT PUZZLE

ACROSS

3. Vein
6. J,K,L,__,O
7. Noise of a bear
8. Liver
10. Oviduct/Eustachian tube
12. Fish egg
13. Kidney
14. Baby or bird noise
17. Mouth
19. Joint
21. English "bye"
23. Body
24. What you kiss with
26. Dine
27. One of *Little Women*
28. Brain
30. Muscle
31. Bone marrow/spinal cord
32. USMC training person
33. Ear
37. Bone
39. Mouth
42. Time measure
43. Biblical character
45. He, she, or ___
46. August birth sign
47. Ovary
50. Curvy letter
51. Unruly crowd
53. Eardrum
54. Stomach

DOWN

1. Intestine
2. Stomach
3. "___ goes the weasel"
4. Ova
5. Bronchus
6. Chairman ___
9. Rectal
11. Nerve
15. Used in a rowboat
16. Rib
18. Gland
19. Artery
20. Testicles
22. Covered with frost
24. On the ___ (criminal)
25. Renal pelvis
29. Cell
32. Teeth
34. Clot (form of)
35. Vessel carrying bile
36. Fat (plural)
38. Oviduct/Eustachian tube
40. Nose
41. Virginian "out"
44. Word of surprise
48. Why you sleep
49. Mouth
51. Muscle
52. ___ else

5. ROOT MULTIPLE CHOICE EXERCISE

Select the correct answer(s) and write the letter(s) of your choice in the space provided.

_____   1. The root for fat is
                 (a) lipo.
                 (b) litho.
                 (c) neuro.
                 (d) none of the above.

_____   2. The rectum is properly called
                 (a) behind.
                 (b) procto.
                 (c) colo.
                 (d) entero.

_____   3. Mast means
                 (a) sail.
                 (b) muscle.
                 (c) breast.
                 (d) chest.

_____   4. The root for ear is
                 (a) ot.
                 (b) oto.
                 (c) oti.
                 (d) all the above.

_____   5. The root for tube is
           (a) vas.
           (b) vaso.
           (c) salpingo.
           (d) oophoro.

_____   6. The root for head is
           (a) psyche.
           (b) cephalo.
           (c) otic.
           (d) ophthalmo.

_____   7. The root for joint is
           (a) osteo.
           (b) arthro.
           (c) rheuma.
           (d) cysto.

_____   8. The root for the loins or abdomen is
           (a) laparo.
           (b) hystero.
           (c) litho.
           (d) lipo.

_____   9. Pertaining to the kidney is
           (a) renal.
           (b) nephro.
           (c) pyelo.
           (d) all of the above.

_____   10. Vas is the root for
           (a) sac.
           (b) vein.
           (c) duct.
           (d) blood.

_____   11.   Adeno is the root for
        (a)   vessel.
        (b)   man.
        (c)   gland.
        (d)   connective tissue.

_____   12.   The root for liver is
        (a)   colpo.
        (b)   hepato.
        (c)   utero.
        (d)   hemato.

_____   13.   Nas is the root for
        (a)   nose.
        (b)   nerve.
        (c)   kidney.
        (d)   none of the above.

_____   14.   Optic is the root for
        (a)   nerve.
        (b)   eye.
        (c)   ovary.
        (d)   mouth.

_____   15.   The root for stone is
        (a)   rocko.
        (b)   litho.
        (c)   lipo.
        (d)   linguo.

_____   16.   Cili is the root for
        (a)   eyelid, small hair, or eyelash.
        (b)   dish made with peppers.
        (c)   cartilage in joints.
        (d)   lips around the mouth.

_____   17.   The proper term for the kidney or renal pelvis is
        (a)   pyelo.
        (b)   cysto.
        (c)   neuro.
        (d)   procto.

_____ 18. Glob is the root for
     (a) the world.
     (b) ball.
     (c) fat.
     (d) tongue.

_____ 19. The root for foot is
     (a) pod.
     (b) ped.
     (c) ortho.
     (d) phleb.

_____ 20. Andr is the root for
     (a) man.
     (b) gland.
     (c) vessel.
     (d) robot.

_____ 21. The root word for nerve is
     (a) fibr.
     (b) angi.
     (c) nephr.
     (d) neuro.

_____ 22. Chondr is the root for
     (a) joint.
     (b) connective tissue.
     (c) tissue.
     (d) cartilage.

_____ 23. The root for mind is
     (a) psych.
     (b) cephal.
     (c) cili.
     (d) pyel.

_____ 24. The root for fungus is
     (a) myc.
     (b) tinea.
     (c) myo.
     (d) muc.

_____ 25. The root for tongue is
  (a) gloss.
  (b) lingu.
  (c) glob.
  (d) salping.

_____ 26. Intercostal means between the
  (a) nose.
  (b) ribs.
  (c) chest.
  (d) cartilage.

_____ 27. Pneumo is the root word for
  (a) breast.
  (b) ribs.
  (c) heart.
  (d) lung.

_____ 28. The root for skin is
  (a) cuti.
  (b) dent.
  (c) hyst.
  (d) derm.

_____ 29. The root for body is
  (a) oophor.
  (b) corpus.
  (c) andro.
  (d) cysto.

_____ 30. The root for intestine is
  (a) gastro.
  (b) colo.
  (c) procto.
  (d) entero.

_____ 31. Angi is the root for
  (a) joint.
  (b) man.
  (c) vessel.
  (d) gland.

_____   32. Blood is the definition of
       (a) cuti.
       (b) hem.
       (c) hist.
       (d) vaso.

_____   33. The root for tissue is
       (a) histo.
       (b) cyto.
       (c) cysto.
       (d) cryo.

_____   34. Gastr is the root for
       (a) colon.
       (b) intestine.
       (c) tongue.
       (d) stomach.

_____   35. The root for eye is
       (a) ocul.
       (b) ophthalm.
       (c) optic.
       (d) all the above.

_____   36. The proper root for the testicle or testis is
       (a) andr.
       (b) colo.
       (c) colpo.
       (d) orchi.

_____   37. The root for bile or gall is
       (a) chol.
       (b) sac.
       (c) cele.
       (d) none of the above.

_____   38. The root for child is
       (a) gyne.
       (b) ped.
       (c) andro.
       (d) none of the above.

_____ 39. The root for vein is

(a) thrombo.

(b) phlebo.

(c) vaso.

(d) hemato.

_____ 40. The root for nose is

(a) neuro.

(b) pharyngo.

(c) rhino.

(d) renal.

_____ 41. The root for chest is

(a) costo.

(b) thoraco.

(c) pneumo.

(d) pectoral.

_____ 42. The root for mucus is

(a) tinea.

(b) muc.

(c) naso.

(d) myo.

_____ 43. Oste is the root for

(a) bone.

(b) eye.

(c) opening, stomach to mouth.

(d) mouth.

_____ 44. The root for kidney is

(a) pyelo.

(b) orchi.

(c) nephro.

(d) salpingo.

_____ 45. Vaso means

(a) tube.

(b) blood vessel, vessel, or duct.

(c) enlargement.

(d) urn.

_____   46. Hyster is the root for
(a) tissue.
(b) liver.
(c) mental illness.
(d) uterus.

_____   47. The root for the heart is
(a) bronch.
(b) cardi.
(c) myo.
(d) enter.

_____   48. The root for cell is
(a) fibro.
(b) cyto.
(c) histo.
(d) cysto.

_____   49. Col is the root for
(a) rib.
(b) colon.
(c) body.
(d) vagina.

_____   50. The root for clot is
(a) thorac.
(b) fibr.
(c) thrombo.
(d) corpus.

_____   51. The root for the bronchus is
(a) lapar.
(b) linguo.
(c) pneumo.
(d) bronch.

_____   52. Hemat is the root for
(a) uterus.
(b) tissue.
(c) liver.
(d) blood.

_____ 53. Chil is the root for
   (a) lip.
   (b) bile.
   (c) fat.
   (d) muscle.

_____ 54. The root for fungus is
   (a) penia.
   (b) tinea.
   (c) fibr.
   (d) orchi.

_____ 55. Myo is the root for
   (a) nose.
   (b) muscle.
   (c) mucus.
   (d) fungus.

_____ 56. The root for horn, cornea, or a corn is
   (a) hernia.
   (b) corpus.
   (c) col.
   (d) kerato.

_____ 57. Procto is the root for
   (a) intestine.
   (b) colon.
   (c) rectum.
   (d) anus.

_____ 58. The root for tooth is
   (a) dontist.
   (b) denti.
   (c) dentine.
   (d) ortho.

_____ 59. The root for connective tissue is
   (a) phlebo.
   (b) fibro.
   (c) histo.
   (d) chondro.

_____   60.   Cryo is the root for
      (a)   eyelid.
      (b)   sac or bladder.
      (c)   rib cage.
      (d)   freeze, cold.

_____   61.   The root for sac or bladder is
      (a)   cysto.
      (b)   colpo.
      (c)   cyto.
      (d)   colo.

INTERNAL ORGANS

6

The most commonly used prefixes, suffixes, and roots pertaining to medicine were covered in Chapters 3, 4, and 5. It is now time to learn basic organ names and placement and to differentiate between the sexes. While the diagram of the male shows the male sexual organs, and the female shows the female sexual organs, *all other organs are the same in both sexes.* The following breakdown merely shows which drawing has which particular organ on it. Most of these terms will not be new ones, as they have already been covered in previous chapters, but they will be reviewed here. Note the similarity between the spelling of **ilium** in the male and **ileum** in the female. **Ilium** is the large pelvic bone; **ileum** is part of the small intestine. One letter can make a big difference.

THE MALE

Root Word/Stem	Meaning
andro	man
arterio	artery
cardio	heart
cephalo	head
chondro	cartilage
costo	rib

THE MALE

Root Word/Stem	Meaning
cysto	bladder
encephalo	brain
ilio	ilium (large pelvic bone)
laparo	abdomen
myelo	bone marrow or spinal cord
myo	muscle
naso	nose
neuro	nerve
nephro	kidney
osteo	bone
orchi	testicle
oro	mouth
phlebo	vein
prostato	prostate
pyelo	pelvis of kidney
rachi	spine
ren	kidney
rhino	nose
sacro	sacrum
stomato	mouth
uretero	ureter
thyro	thyroid
thoraco	chest

THE FEMALE

Root Word/Stem	Meaning
ano	anus
append	appendix
broncho	bronchus
chole	bile
cholecysto	gallbladder (chole = bile; cysto = bladder)
choledocho	bile duct (docho = duct)

THE FEMALE

Root Word/Stem	Meaning
colo	large intestine
colpo	vagina
cranio	skull
denti, dont	teeth
derma	skin
entero	small intestine
esophago	esophagus
gastro	stomach
glosso, linguo	tongue
gyn, gyne, gyneco	woman
hept, hepato	liver
hystero	uterus
ileo	ileum (division of small intestine)
masto	breast
metro	uterus
oculo	eye
oophor	ovary
ophthalmo	eye
otic	ear
oto	ear
procto	rectum
pharyngo	pharynx
pneumo	lung
salpingo	oviduct or Eustachian tube
tracheo	trachea

The following pages contain line drawings of the male and the female, with each organ or area identified, as it is listed in the previous tables. While *neuro* (nerve) is shown in the male head, nerves are found in all parts of the body. The same holds true for *myo* (muscle), *osteo* (bone), *arthro* (joint), *arterio* (artery), *mast* (breast), *phlebo* (vein), and so on. Also, only one of each organ is shown, although there are two eyes, ears, ovaries, more than one tooth, and so on.

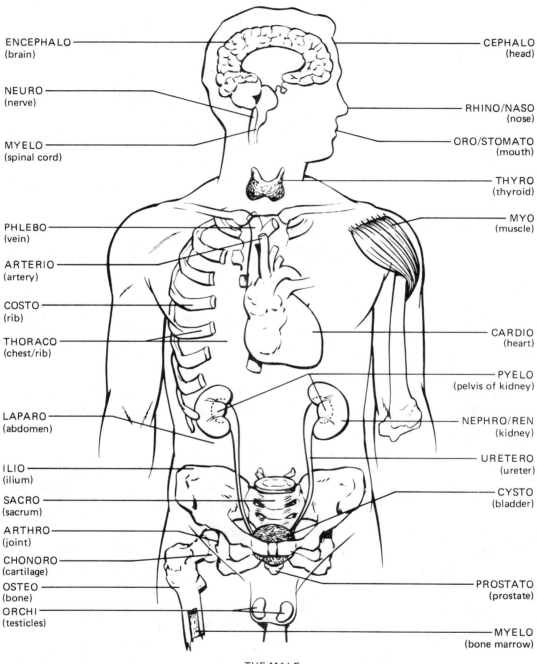

ENCEPHALO
(brain)

NEURO
(nerve)

MYELO
(spinal cord)

PHLEBO
(vein)

ARTERIO
(artery)

COSTO
(rib)

THORACO
(chest/rib)

LAPARO
(abdomen)

ILIO
(ilium)

SACRO
(sacrum)

ARTHRO
(joint)

CHONORO
(cartilage)

OSTEO
(bone)

ORCHI
(testicles)

CEPHALO
(head)

RHINO/NASO
(nose)

ORO/STOMATO
(mouth)

THYRO
(thyroid)

MYO
(muscle)

CARDIO
(heart)

PYELO
(pelvis of kidney)

NEPHRO/REN
(kidney)

URETERO
(ureter)

CYSTO
(bladder)

PROSTATO
(prostate)

MYELO
(bone marrow)

THE MALE
ANDRO (man)

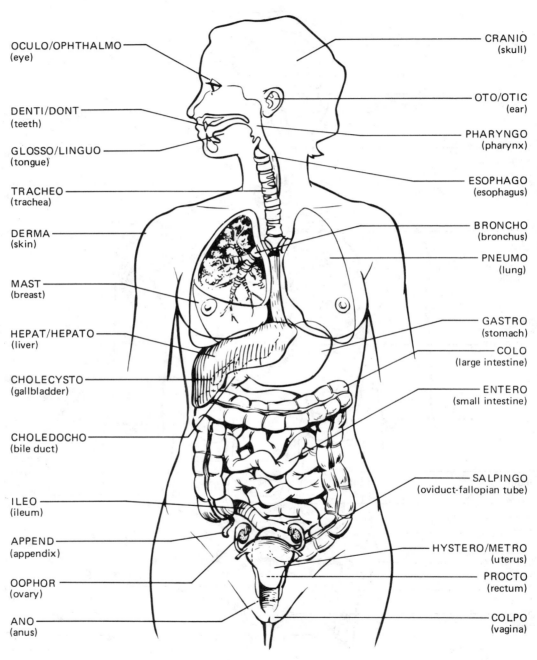

OCULO/OPHTHALMO
(eye)

CRANIO
(skull)

DENTI/DONT
(teeth)

OTO/OTIC
(ear)

GLOSSO/LINGUO
(tongue)

PHARYNGO
(pharynx)

TRACHEO
(trachea)

ESOPHAGO
(esophagus)

DERMA
(skin)

BRONCHO
(bronchus)

MAST
(breast)

PNEUMO
(lung)

HEPAT/HEPATO
(liver)

GASTRO
(stomach)

CHOLECYSTO
(gallbladder)

COLO
(large intestine)

CHOLEDOCHO
(bile duct)

ENTERO
(small intestine)

ILEO
(ileum)

SALPINGO
(oviduct-fallopian tube)

APPEND
(appendix)

HYSTERO/METRO
(uterus)

OOPHOR
(ovary)

PROCTO
(rectum)

ANO
(anus)

COLPO
(vagina)

THE FEMALE
GYNE (woman)

Careful study of these drawings will provide a general idea of the location of an organ as well as which *quadrant* it is located in. This aids in locating and understanding terms used to identify an area, such as right upper quadrant, left upper quadrant, and so on.

1. INTERNAL ORGAN MATCHING EXERCISE

The terms on the left pertain to internal anatomy. Match the component in the left column with the correct definition in the right column. Place the letter of the definition in the provided space.

_____	1. cardio	a.	joint
_____	2. gastro	b.	eardrum
_____	3. myelo	c.	brain
_____	4. cholecysto	d.	ilium or flank
_____	5. nephro	e.	pleura, side or rib
_____	6. procto	f.	bone marrow—spinal cord
_____	7. myringo	g.	heart
_____	8. salpingo	h.	gland
_____	9. broncho	i.	fallopian tube
_____	10. ilio	j.	intestinal tract
_____	11. hepato	k.	gallbladder
_____	12. arthro	l.	artery
_____	13. pyelo	m.	kidney
_____	14. ileo	n.	bone
_____	15. costo	o.	liver
_____	16. Neuro	p.	vein
_____	17. pleuro	q.	pelvis of kidney
_____	18. oophoro	r.	ileum
_____	19. encephalo	s.	bronchus
_____	20. osteo	t.	nerve
_____	21. adeno	u.	stomach
_____	22. phlebo	v.	ovary
_____	23. orchio	w.	anus, rectum
_____	24. entero	x.	rib
_____	25. arterio	y.	testis

2. INTERNAL ORGAN PUZZLE

ACROSS

2. Trachea
4. Bone marrow/spinal cord
7. Lung
8. Appendix
10. Small intestine
11. Liver
13. Chest
17. He, she, or _____
19. Yield or grant
20. From, away
22. Spinal cord/bone marrow
23. Nerve
24. Tough nut (abbr.)
25a. Vein
27. Esophagus
30. Bile duct
32. Sound of laughter
33. Eye
34. Bull-ring cheer
36. Mouth
42. Inferior (position)
43. Storage room above house
44. Oviduct or Eustachian tube
47. Brain
50. Mouth
51. Emergency room
52. Muscle
54. Anus
56. Post office
57. Spanish gold
60. Nose

61. Joint
62. Alkaline balance
63. Plural nose
64. Thyroid
66. Writing instrument
68. Large intestine
69. Long period of time
70. Rib
72. Stomach
73. Uterus
74. Eye
78. Tooth
80. Testicles
81. Abdomen
82. Mouth

DOWN

1. Skin
2. A preposition
3. Liver
5. Woman
6. Ureters
8. Artery
9. Rectum
12. Prostate
14. Kidney
15. Near
16. Head
17. Intestine, ileum
18. Anus
20. Entirety

21. Honey maker
22. Cow sound
25d. Santa saying
26. Before daylight
28. Ear
29. Tongue
30. Gallbladder
31. Skull
35. Female sheep
36. Sacrum, sacroiliac
37. Ovary
38. Over six feet is _____
39. Ear
40. Bladder
41. Bile duct
42. Bronchus
44. Cartilage
46. Pharynx
48. Kidney
49. Heart
52. Breast
53. Vagina
55. Bile
58. Blood factor
59. Piggy noise
62. Renal pelvis of kidney
65. Combining form
67. Uterus
71. Tattled
75. Ear
76. Ilium
77. Man
79. Small intestine

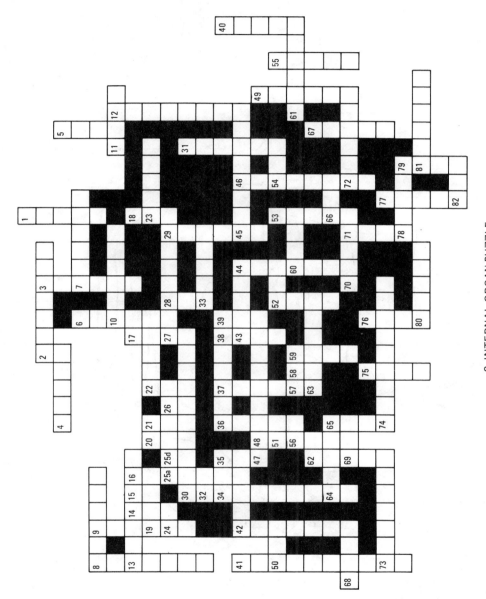

2. INTERNAL ORGAN PUZZLE

135

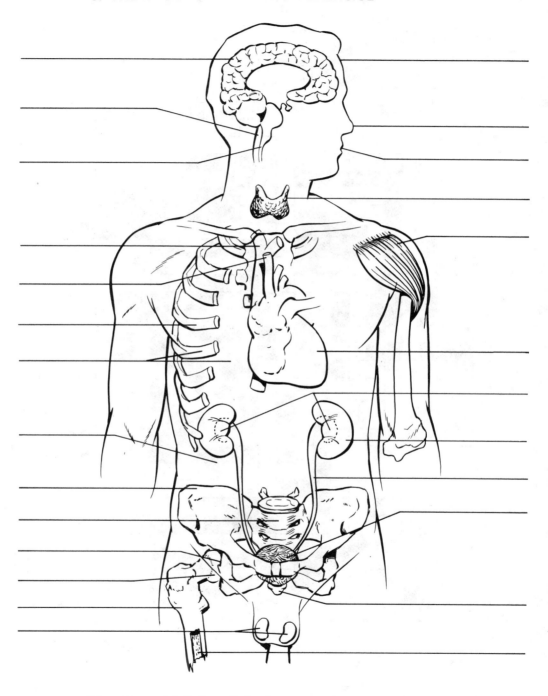

Identify and label each body part of this male figure.

4. THE FEMALE IDENTIFICATION EXERCISE

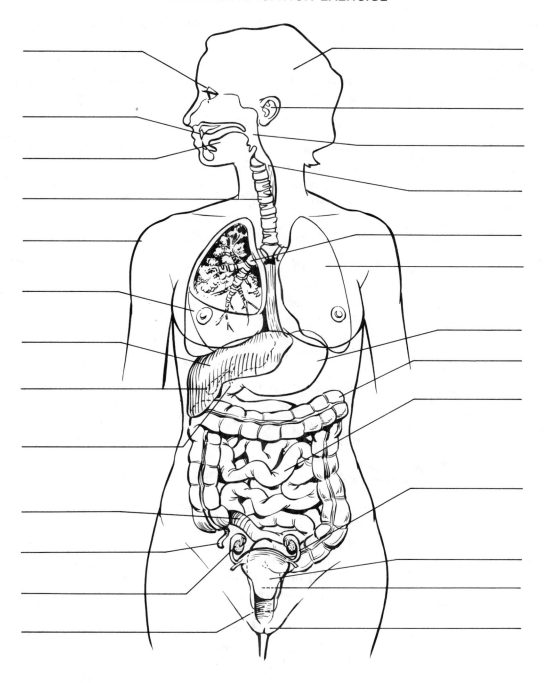

Identify and label each body part of this female figure.

5. INTERNAL ORGAN MULTIPLE CHOICE EXERCISE

Select the correct answer(s), and write the letter(s) of your choice in the space provided.

_____   1.   Rachi is
     (a)   an instrument of torture.
     (b)   spine.
     (c)   spinal cord.
     (d)   all of the above.
     (e)   none of the above.

_____   2.   Thoraco means
     (a)   chest.
     (b)   breast.
     (c)   thyroid.
     (d)   all of the above.
     (e)   none of the above.

_____   3.   The word for liver is
     (a)   hepato.
     (b)   encephalo.
     (c)   nephro.
     (d)   all of the above.
     (e)   none of the above.

_____   4.   Encephalo means
     (a)   within the hair.
     (b)   within the skull.
     (c)   within the brain.
     (d)   all of the above.
     (e)   none of the above.

_____   5.   Choledocho means
     (a)   bile duct or tube.
     (b)   liver duct or tube.
     (c)   egg duct or tube.
     (d)   all of the above.
     (e)   none of the above.

_____   6. Ureto refers to

    (a) joint.

    (b) artery.

    (c) man.

    (d) all of the above.

    (e) none of the above.

_____   7. Oste means

    (a) mouth.

    (b) ureter.

    (c) bone.

    (d) all of the above.

    (e) none of the above.

_____   8. The word uterus means

    (a) womb.

    (b) hystero.

    (c) metro.

    (d) all of the above.

    (e) none of the above.

_____   9. The large intestine is called

    (a) laparo.

    (b) gastro.

    (c) colo.

    (d) all of the above.

    (e) none of the above.

_____   10. Colpo is

    (a) colon.

    (b) vagina.

    (c) rib.

    (d) all of the above.

    (e) none of the above.

_____   11. Heart is termed

    (a) cardio.

    (b) costo.

    (c) thoraco.

    (d) all of the above.

    (e) none of the above.

_____   12.   Myo means
     (a)   bone marrow.
     (b)   muscle.
     (c)   spinal cord.
     (d)   all of the above.
     (e)   none of the above.

_____   13.   The large pelvic bone is called
     (a)   illeo.
     (b)   ilio.
     (c)   ileo.
     (d)   all of the above.
     (e)   none of the above.

_____   14.   Prostato means
     (a)   vein.
     (b)   prostate.
     (c)   on your face.
     (d)   all of the above.
     (e)   none of the above.

_____   15.   Broncho means
     (a)   stomach.
     (b)   mouth.
     (c)   abdomen.
     (d)   all of the above.
     (e)   none of the above.

_____   16.   Orchi means
     (a)   prostate.
     (b)   testicles.
     (c)   ovary.
     (d)   all of the above.
     (e)   none of the above.

_____   17.   The oviduct is also called
     (a)   fallopian tube.
     (b)   salpingo.
     (c)   egg passage or tube.
     (d)   all of the above.
     (e)   none of the above.

_____ 18. The word for intestine is
    (a) illeo.
    (b) ilio.
    (c) ileo.
    (d) all of the above.
    (e) none of the above.

_____ 19. The word for eye is
    (a) otic.
    (b) oto.
    (c) ophthalmo.
    (d) all of the above.
    (e) none of the above.

_____ 20. Derma means
    (a) outer.
    (b) hard.
    (c) skin.
    (d) all of the above.
    (e) none of the above.

_____ 21. Man is
    (a) arterio.
    (b) arthro.
    (c) ano.
    (d) all of the above.
    (e) none of the above.

_____ 22. Myelo means
    (a) bone marrow.
    (b) muscle.
    (c) spinal cord.
    (d) all of the above.
    (e) none of the above.

_____ 23. Ano means
    (a) appendix.
    (b) man.
    (c) anus.
    (d) all of the above.
    (e) none of the above.

_____ 24. The word for nerve is
  (a) nephro.
  (b) naso.
  (c) nevoid.
  (d) all of the above.
  (e) none of the above.

_____ 25. The word for artery is
  (a) arterio.
  (b) arthro.
  (c) phlebo.
  (d) all of the above.
  (e) none of the above.

_____ 26. Gyne is
  (a) woman.
  (b) female.
  (c) feminine.
  (d) all of the above.
  (e) none of the above.

_____ 27. The word for nose is
  (a) scento.
  (b) rhino.
  (c) naso.
  (d) all of the above.
  (e) none of the above.

_____ 28. The stomach is
  (a) laparo.
  (b) gastro.
  (c) colo.
  (d) all of the above.
  (e) none of the above.

_____ 29. Chondro is
  (a) the colon.
  (b) muscle.
  (c) cartilage.
  (d) all of the above.
  (e) none of the above.

_____ 30. Which of the following refer to the kidney?

    (a) ren.

    (b) nephro.

    (c) renal.

    (d) all of the above.

    (e) none of the above.

_____ 31. Cranio means

    (a) encephalo.

    (b) skull.

    (c) cephalo.

    (d) all of the above.

    (e) none of the above.

_____ 32. Cholecysto means

    (a) gall duct.

    (b) urinary bladder.

    (c) gall bladder.

    (d) all of the above.

    (e) none of the above.

_____ 33. Cephalo is

    (a) cartilage.

    (b) skull.

    (c) head.

    (d) all of the above.

    (e) none of the above.

_____ 34. The small intestine is termed

    (a) gastro.

    (b) entero.

    (c) colo.

    (d) all of the above.

    (e) none of the above.

_____ 35. Andro means

    (a) joint.

    (b) artery.

    (c) man.

    (d) all of the above.

    (e) none of the above.

_____ 36. Joint is
   (a) andro.
   (b) arterio.
   (c) arthro.
   (d) all of the above.
   (e) none of the above.

_____ 37. Phlebo means
   (a) nerve.
   (b) kidney.
   (c) vein.
   (d) all of the above.
   (e) none of the above.

_____ 38. Pyelo means
   (a) hemorrhoids.
   (b) pelvis of kidney.
   (c) rectum.
   (d) all of the above.
   (e) none of the above.

_____ 39. The word for kidney is
   (a) nephro.
   (b) neuro.
   (c) cysto.
   (d) all of the above.
   (e) none of the above.

_____ 40. Mouth is
   (a) oro.
   (b) os.
   (c) stomato.
   (d) all of the above.
   (e) none of the above.

_____ 41. Bone marrow is
   (a) myco.
   (b) muco.
   (c) myelo.
   (d) all of the above.
   (e) none of the above.

_____ 42. The heart (cardio) is located in the
   (a) abdominal cavity.
   (b) head cavity.
   (c) chest cavity.
   (d) all of the above.
   (e) none of the above.

_____ 43. Hepato means
   (a) bone marrow.
   (b) muscle.
   (c) uterus.
   (d) all of the above.
   (e) none of the above.

_____ 44. The root mast means
   (a) chest.
   (b) breast.
   (c) thyroid.
   (d) all of the above.
   (e) none of the above.

_____ 45. Stomato is
   (a) stomach.
   (b) mouth.
   (c) abdomen.
   (d) all of the above.
   (e) none of the above.

_____ 46. Cysto means
   (a) rib.
   (b) bladder.
   (c) cartilage.
   (d) all of the above.
   (e) none of the above.

_____ 47. Sacro means
   (a) sacrum.
   (b) sacred.
   (c) skull.
   (d) all of the above.
   (e) none of the above.

_____ 48. Rhino means
  (a) skin.
  (b) large.
  (c) nose.
  (d) all of the above.
  (e) none of the above.

_____ 49. Rib is
  (a) costo.
  (b) cardio.
  (c) chondro.
  (d) all of the above.
  (e) none of the above.

_____ 50. The abdomen is
  (a) laparo.
  (b) appendo.
  (c) gastro.
  (d) all of the above.
  (e) none of the above.

_____ 51. Thyro means
  (a) trachea.
  (b) chest.
  (c) thyroid.
  (d) all of the above.
  (e) none of the above.

_____ 52. The appendix is
  (a) colo.
  (b) append.
  (c) ileo.
  (d) all of the above.
  (e) none of the above.

_____ 53. Neuro means
  (a) nerve.
  (b) artery.
  (c) vein.
  (d) all of the above.
  (e) none of the above.

_____ 54. The word for skull is
   (a) cephalo.
   (b) cranio.
   (c) encephalo.
   (d) all of the above.
   (e) none of the above.

_____ 55. The word for bile duct is
   (a) choledocho.
   (b) cholecysto.
   (c) cholesalpingo.
   (d) all of the above.
   (e) none of the above.

_____ 56. Procto means
   (a) prostate.
   (b) kidney.
   (c) rectum.
   (d) all of the above.
   (e) none of the above.

_____ 57. Broncho means
   (a) bronchus.
   (b) a wild horse.
   (c) bladder.
   (d) all of the above.
   (e) none of the above.

PUTTING IT ALL
TOGETHER

7

At this point, you are ready to utilize the knowledge you have gained from the previous chapters. This chapter consists of a variety of exercises using the prefixes, suffixes, roots, locations, positions, and anatomy covered, as well as some new terms (which can be found in any comprehensive medical dictionary). You will also have an opportunity to "create" words, using the bits and pieces of words you know.

Now is also the time for you to utilize a medical dictionary. Should you run across a word piece you are unfamiliar with, you should be able to make an educated guess as to where it is located, what system it is in, what specialty it applies to, or if it is a surgical or diagnostic term.

At the completion of this chapter, you should be able to read, pronounce, and understand a wide variety of medical reports, papers, and dictation. You will also be able to use a medical dictionary for spelling checks, and will find your spelling and vocabulary constantly improving.

A helpful idea is to highlight a word the first time it is looked up in the dictionary to verify spelling. If the source is consulted again for the same word, the word is obviously one used fairly often and one you have difficulty spelling. Enter its proper spelling on a list kept near your workplace; when you no longer need to check the spelling of the word, you can delete it from your list.

1. REVIEW DEFINITION EXERCISE

Define each component and then define the entire word.

1. post_____ partum_____

   postpartum = _____

2. dys_____ pep_____ sia_____

   dyspepsia = _____

3. audio_____ meter_____

   audiometer = _____

4. pneumo_____ centesis_____

   pneumocentesis = _____

5. a_____ phas_____ ia_____

   aphasia = _____

6. procto_____ ptosis_____

   proctoptosis = _____

7. hemo_____ stasis_____

   hemostasis = _____

8. hernio_____ rrhaphy_____

   herniorrhaphy = _____

9. micro_____ scope_____

   microscope = _____

10. oophor_____ectomy_____

    oophorectomy = _____

11. metro_____rrhagia_____

    metrorrhagia = _____

12. crypt_____orchid_____ism_____

    cryptorchidism (cryptorchism) = _____

13. dipl_____opia_____

    diplopia = _____

14. necr_____ops_____

    necropsy = _____

15. hyper_____troph_____

    hypertrophy = _____

16. sub_____ cutane_____ ous_____

    subcutaneous = _____

17. endo_____card_____ium_____

    endocardium = _____

18. trans_____mit_____

    transmit = _____

19. hyster_____ectomy_____

    hysterectomy = _____

20. hepat_____itis_____

    hepatitis = _____

21. hemi_____an_____esthesia_____

    hemianesthesia = _____

22. quadr_____plegia_____

    quadriplegia = _____

23. gastro_____scope_____

    gastroscope = _____

24. macro_____glossia_____

    macroglossia = _____

25. dent_____algia_____

    dentalgia = _____

2. REVIEW DEFINITION EXERCISE

Define each component and then define the entire word.

1. peri_____metrium_____

    perimetrium = _____

2. epi_____cyst_____itis_____

    epicystitis = _____

3. micro_____cardia_____

microcardia = _____

4. dys_____pnea_____

dyspnea = _____

5. hypo_____thermia_____

hypothermia = _____

6. leuco_____derma_____

leucoderma = _____

7. hystero_____my_____oma_____

hysteromyoma = _____

8. hyper_____algia_____

hyperalgia = _____

9. neuro_____genic_____

neurogenic = _____

10. histo_____pathology_____

histopathology = _____

11. thorac_____ostomy_____

thoracostomy = _____

12. hemat_____oma_____

hematoma = _____

13. psycho_____ path _____

psychopath = _____

14. gastro_____ scopy _____

gastroscopy = _____

15. gastro_____ ptosis _____

gastroptosis = _____

16. chole_____ cysto_____ gram _____

cholecystogram = _____

17. hyper_____ esthesia _____

hyperesthesia = _____

18. nephr_____ otomy _____

nephrotomy = _____

19. pharyng_____ itis _____

pharyngitis = _____

20. nephro_____ lith_____ osis _____

nephrolithosis = _____

21. chole_____ cyst_____ ectomy _____

cholecystectomy = _____

22. my_____ oma _____

myoma = _____

23.   osteo_____scler_____osis_____

osteosclerosis = _____

24.   arthr_____ectomy_____

arthrectomy = _____

25.   noct_____ambulism_____

noctambulism = _____

3. REVIEW DEFINITION EXERCISE

Define each component and then define the entire word.

1.   opisth_____ otic_____

opisthotic = _____

2.   necro_____phobia_____

necrophobia = _____

3.   psycho_____genic_____

psychogenic = _____

4.   angio_____card_____itis_____

angiocarditis = _____

5.   tachy_____card_____

tachycardia = _____

6. cyan_____ osis_____

 cyanosis = _____

7. melan_____ oma_____

 melanoma = _____

8. hemat_____ emesis_____

 hematemesis = _____

9. dys_____ meno_____ rrhea_____

 dysmenorrhea = _____

10. osteo_____ arthr_____ itis_____

 osteoarthritis = _____

11. hemo_____ pneumo_____ thorax_____

 hemopneumothorax = _____

12. cardio_____ peri_____ pexy_____

 cardiopericardiopexy = _____

13. inter_____ costal_____

 intercostal = _____

14. osteo_____ myel_____ itis_____

 osteomyelitis = _____

15. masto_____ pexy_____

 mastopexy = _____

16. sub_____costal_____

    subcostal = _____

17. gyneco_____logist_____

    gynecologist = _____

18. poly_____uria_____

    polyuria = _____

19. pneumon_____itis_____

    pneumonitis = _____

20. tetra_____plegia_____

    tetraplegia = _____

21. chole_____lith_____osis_____

    cholelithosis = _____

22. hemat_____uria_____

    hematuria = _____

23. pyo_____genic_____

    pyogenic = _____

24. retro_____lingual_____

    retrolingual = _____

25. gluco_____genic_____

    glucogenic = _____

4. REVIEW DEFINITION EXERCISE

Define each component and then define the entire word.

1. mono_____ neural_____

   mononeural = _____

2. phago_____ cyt_____ osis_____

   phagocytosis = _____

3. lipo_____ derm_____

   lipodermia = _____

4. path_____ ology_____

   pathology = _____

5. taxi_____ dermy_____

   taxidermy = _____

6. oto_____ scope_____

   otoscope = _____

7. neo_____ natal_____

   neonatal = _____

8. anti_____ pyretic_____

   antipyretic = _____

9. ante_____ partum_____

   antepartum = _____

10. hydro_____cele_____

    hydrocele = _____

11. ex_____cise_____

    excise = _____

12. ovi_____duct_____

    oviduct = _____

13. hypo_____glyc_____emia_____

    hypoglycemia = _____

14. hystero_____pexy_____

    hysteropexy = _____

15. arterio_____scler_____osis_____

    arteriosclerosis = _____

16. endo_____scopy_____

    endoscopy = _____

17. myc_____ology_____

    mycology = _____

18. histo_____gram_____

    histogram = _____

19. neuro_____pathic_____

    neuropathic = _____

20. crypt_____orchid_____ectomy_____

    cryptorchidectomy = _____

21. nephro_____lith_____iasis_____

    nephrolithiasis = _____

22. phleb_____itis_____

    phlebitis = _____

23. thrombo_____phleb_____itis_____

    thrombophlebitis = _____

24. vas_____ectomy_____

    vasectomy = _____

25. pneumon_____itis_____

    pneumonitis = _____

5. PUTTING IT ALL TOGETHER PUZZLE

ACROSS

2. Difficult breathing
4. Double vision
6. Between the ribs
8. After birth
11. Surgical removal of ovary
13. Dry mouth
15. Hidden or undescended testicle
17. Inflammation of a joint
18. Agent to check escape of blood
19. Above the kidney
20. Nourishment
22. Slow heart

DOWN

1. Inflammation of a joint
2. Difficult or painful digestion
3. Surgical incision of a vein
5. Fallen rectum
7. Scanty urine
8. Puncture of and removal or withdrawal of fluid from lung
9. Uterine bleeding
10. Autopsy
12. Blood making
14. Between the ribs
16. Eating or destruction of cells
21. Absence or lack of speech

160

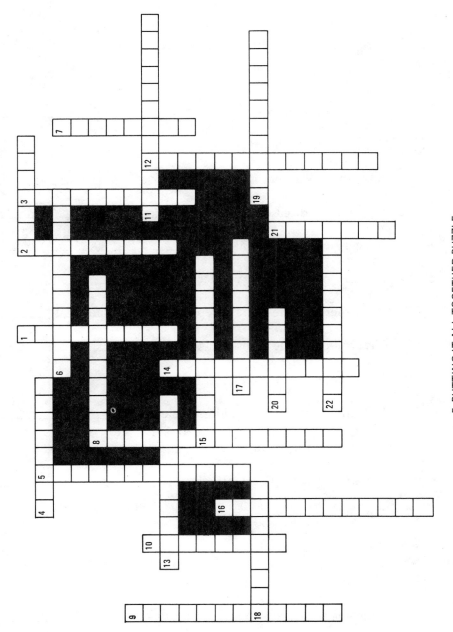

5. PUTTING IT ALL TOGETHER PUZZLE

6. REVIEW COMPLETION EXERCISE

Fill in the blanks with the name of the proper medical or surgical specialty.

1. Surgery on children _____

2. Surgery on the heart _____

3. Surgery on the nervous system _____

4. Surgery on diseases of the mouth _____

5. Surgery on the skeletal system _____

6. Surgery on the urinary tract _____

7. Treatment of the female reproductive system _____

8. Treatment of the mind _____

9. Treatment of the aged _____

10. Treatment of cancers/malignancies _____

11. Treatment for asthma _____

12. Treatment for a heart attack _____

13. One who puts you to sleep _____

14. Treatment of eyes _____

15. Treatment of a blood disease _____

16. Treatment of the stomach/intestines _____

17. Treatment of diseases of the rectum _____

18. Treatment of overall health _____

19. Treatment of the skin _____

20. Treatment of infertility in men _____

21. Counseling for inherited diseases _____

22. Treatment of hormonal problems _____

23. Treatment of pregnancy/delivery _____

24. X-rays and diagnostics _____

25. Filling of a prescription _____

7. REVIEW COMPLETION EXERCISE

Fill in the blank with the word that most correctly completes the sentence.

1. Posterior means the same as _____ .

2. A disease or infection in the blood is _____ .

3. Inflammation of the heart from within is _____ .

4. Angionecrosis is _____ .

5. A very fast heartbeat is _____ .

6. Meningitis is _____ .

7. The outer layer of skin is called the _____ .

8. Inflamed skin is called _____ .

9. A condition of blood in the oviduct is called _____

    _____ .

10. The surgical removal of the gallbladder is _____ .

11. Water or fluid in a hernia or sac is _____ .

12. A ruptured uterus is a _____ .

13. Hormones are secreted by which system? _____ .

14. Water on the brain is _____ .

15. Rachicentesis means _____ .

16. Sleep seizure, or an uncontrollable desire to sleep, is called

_____ .

17. Nail eating (or biting) is _____ onychosis .

18. An abnormal fear of heights is _____ .

19. The study of the inside of the brain is _____ .

20. Upon the skin is _____ .

21. Behind the sternum, or breastbone, is _____ .

22. To be partly, or about half, awake is to be _____ .

23. Thin-skinned is _____ .

24. If you are supine, you are _____ .

25. Pertaining to the back of the body is _____ .

8. REVIEW DEFINITION EXERCISE

Read the following sentences or paragraphs and then write an explanation of what you have read by defining italicized words, then paraphrasing the passage.

1. *Diagnostic impression:* Extensive *diverticulosis* and focal *diverticulitis*, with intramural abscess formation, was found in the sigmoid colon.

    diverticulosis: _____

    diverticulitis: _____

    _____

    _____

    _____

2. *Surgery:* Exploratory *laparotomy*, colon *resection*.

    laparotomy: _____

    resection: _____

    _____

    _____

    _____

3. Under general *anesthesia*, the patient was prepped and draped. The abdomen was entered through a *lower midline* incision.

    anesthesia: _____

    lower midline: _____

    _____

    _____

    _____

4. On entering the *peritoneal cavity*, there were a few *adhesions* to the *anterior* abdominal wall, which were divided. . . . The right *hepatic* lobe was difficult to examine because of *adhesions*.

    peritoneal: _____

cavity: _____

adhesions: _____

anterior: _____

hepatic: _____

_____

_____

_____

_____

5. Spleen was grossly normal to *palpation.* . . . There was *inflammation* about the sigmoid colon and it was *adherent* to the *lateral pelvic* wall.

palpation: _____

inflammation: _____

adherent: _____

lateral: _____

pelvic: _____

_____

_____

_____

_____

6. The *ureter* on the left side was . . . in the course of the *dissection*. Mesentery of the colon was divided and ligated with 2-0 silk ties. Approximately 12 inches of sigmoid colon was removed and two-layered 3-0 silk *anastomosis* was carried out.

    ureter: _____

    dissection: _____

    anastomosis: _____

    _____

    _____

    _____

    _____

7. An elliptical incision was used to perform a modified radical *mastectomy.Dissection* was carried *medially* through the *sternal* borders, *superiorly* to the *infraclavicular* area, *laterally* to the latissimus dorsi and *inferiorly* to the insertion of the rectus muscle. . . . Two catheters were left in the *subcutaneous* area and brought out through the skin.

    mastectomy: _____

    dissection: _____

    medially: _____

    sternal: _____

    superiorly: _____

    infraclavicular: _____

    laterally: _____

inferiorly: _____

subcutaneous: _____

_____

_____

_____

_____

_____

_____

_____

_____

8. A section of the *posterior* surface of the breast shows *hemorrhagic fibroadipose* tissue and some skeletal muscle.

posterior: _____

hemorrhagic: _____

fibroadipose: _____

_____

_____

9. Twenty *axillary* lymph node sections from all four *quadrants* are examined and are negative for *metastatic carcinoma*. These nodes show only benign sinus *histiocytosis* and follicular *hyperplasia*.

axillary: _____

quadrants: _____

metastatic: _____

carcinoma: _____

histiocytosis: _____

hyperplasia: _____

_____

_____

_____

_____

_____

10. Examination of numerous sections from the *mastectomy* reveals
     interlobular sclerosis, *duct ectasia*, focal *adenosis*, and *sclerosing*
     adenosis. The skin lesion reveals a compound nevus with most
     of the cells within the *dermis*. Some *keratin* tunnels are noted in
     this lesion.

mastectomy: _____

interlobular: _____

sclerosis: _____

duct: _____

ectasia: _____

adenosis: _____

sclerosing: _____

dermis: _____

keratin: _____

_____

_____

_____

_____

_____

_____

_____

11. Procedure: Exploratory *laparotomy, proximal colostomy,* and mucous fistula:

laparotomy: _____

proximal: _____

colostomy: _____

_____

_____

_____

9. REVIEW DEFINITION EXERCISE

Read each passage and write the proper medical equivalents for the lay terms listed. Then write a short descriptive medical summary of the paragraph using medical terminology.

1. The victim had cold, blue skin; very rapid heartbeat; and pain in the body.

    Cold, blue skin: _____

    Very rapid heartbeat: _____

    Pain in the body: _____

    _____

    _____

    _____

2. Symptoms included uncontrolled restlessness, excessive thirst, vomited or coughed-up blood, and blood in the urine:

    Excessive thirst: _____

    Vomited or coughed-up blood: _____

    Blood in the urine: _____

    _____

    _____

    _____

3. After a head injury, the patient had a rapid flow of blood from the nose and throat, loss of feeling, paralysis of one side of the body, a slow heartbeat, and vomiting of blood.

    Rapid flow of blood: _____

    Nose and throat: _____

    Loss of feeling: _____

    Paralysis of one side of the body: _____

    Slow heartbeat: _____

Vomiting of blood: _____

_____

_____

_____

_____

_____

4.   The nosebleed came from high blood pressure and failure of the blood to clot.

Nosebleed: new word—epistaxis _____

High blood pressure: _____

Failure of the blood to clot: _____

_____

_____

_____

10. REVIEW DEFINITION EXERCISE

Explain each operative procedure listed below.

1.   colostomy closure: _____

_____

2. tubal anastomosis-laparoscopy: _____

_____

3. exploratory laparotomy: _____

_____

4. tympanomastoidectomy: _____

_____

5. microsuspension laryngoscopy: _____

_____

6. adenoidectomy: _____

_____

7. cystoscopy: _____

_____

8. right retrograde pyelogram: _____

_____

9. excision peritoneal lesions: _____

_____

10. palatoplasty: _____

_____

11. parotidectomy: _____

_____

12. colocystectomy: _____

_____

13. subtemporal/suboccipital craniotomy resection: _____

_____

14. segmental mastectomy, possible lymph node biopsy: _____

_____

15. costoscopy, bilateral and retrograde: _____

_____

16. colonoscopy: _____

_____

17. lid blepharoplasty: _____

_____

18. cholecystectomy: _____

_____

19. bilateral adenoidectomy: _____

_____

20. tonsillectomy: _____

_____

21. left medial epicondylectomy: _____

_____

22. septoplasty: _____

_____

23. hydrocelectomy: _____

_____

24. urethrolithotomy: _____

_____

25. arthroscopy: _____

_____

POSTTEST

Match the word parts in the left column with definitions in the right column.

Part A

_____	1. mit	a.	breath
_____	2. odes	b.	breathing
_____	3. ole	c.	constriction, compression
_____	4. otomy	d.	cutting, incision
_____	5. scopy	e.	disease
_____	6. ule	f.	dropping of an organ
_____	7. pathy	g.	education, child
_____	8. oda	h.	examine, observation
_____	9. rrhaphy	i.	form, resemblance, like
_____	10. stalsis	j.	giving birth to
_____	11. ology	k.	hard
_____	12. ptosis	l.	like, resemblance
_____	13. oid	m.	like, resemblance
_____	14. sclero	n.	opening into, communication between

_____ 15. oma   o. process/condition of, disease, act of

_____ 16. osis   p. sent, full of

_____ 17. phag   q. small

_____ 18. parous   r. small

_____ 19. pnea   s. spitting, saliva

_____ 20. sophy   t. study of, science of

_____ 21. spire   u. suture, repair

_____ 22. tropic   v. swallow, eating

_____ 23. stomy   w. tumor, growth

_____ 24. pedia   x. too few

_____ 25. penia   y. turning toward, tending to turn/change

_____ 26. ptysis   z. wisdom, art, skill

Part B

_____ 27. phobia   a. abnormal fear of, dread

_____ 28. taxis   b. anything formed

_____ 29. trophy   c. anything formed

_____ 30. plasm   d. arrangement

_____ 31. pod   e. blood vessel, vessel

_____ 32. ped   f. cell

_____ 33. plast   g. chest

_____ 34. osis   h. child, foot

_____ 35. tomy   i. clot

_____ 36. uria   j. cutting, incision

_____ 37. adeno   k. foot

_____ 38. vaso   l. fungus

_____ 39. cyto   m. gland

_____ 40. histo   n. in the urine

_____ 41. myo   o. liver

_____ 42. thoraco   p. marrow, spinal cord

_____ 43. procto   q. muscle

_____ 44. salpingo   r. nose

_____	45.	myelo	s. nourishment
_____	46.	myco	t. ovary
_____	47.	pyelo	u. process, condition of, disease
_____	48.	rhino, naso	v. rectum
_____	49.	oophoro	w. renal pelvis, pelvis of kidney
_____	50.	thrombo	x. skin
_____	51.	derma	y. tissue
_____	52.	hepato	z. tube

Part C

_____	53.	entero	a. blood vessel
_____	54.	orchi	b. bone
_____	55.	cardio	c. breast
_____	56.	mast	d. connective tissue
_____	57.	renal	e. ear
_____	58.	gastro	f. eye
_____	59.	oculo/ ophthalmo	g. fat
_____	60.	psyche	h. heart
_____	61.	neuro	i. intestine
_____	62.	arthro	j. joint
_____	63.	angio	k. kidney
_____	64.	costo	l. lung, air
_____	65.	nephro	m. mind
_____	66.	phlebo, ven(a, o)	n. mucus
_____	67.	ot	o. nerve
_____	68.	fibro	p. pertaining to kidney
_____	69.	hystero	q. rib
_____	70.	cysto	r. sac, bladder
_____	71.	osteo	s. stomach
_____	72.	muco	t. testicle
_____	73.	lipo	u. uterus
_____	74.	pneumo	v. vein

Fill in the blanks.

75. Retrolingual means _____ the

   _____ .

76. Anesthesia means lack of _____ .

77. Mononeural means one _____ .

78. Hypotension means _____
   pressure.

79. Polyuria means _____
   urination.

80. Cyanosis means a _____ of

   being _____ .

81. Intravenous means _____ a

   _____ .

82. Excise means to _____ .

83. Malnutrition means nutrition which is _____ .

84. Glucogenic means _____ by
   sugar.

85. Macroencephaly means a large _____ .

86. Megacolon means a _____

   which is _____ .

87. Necrophobia means an _____

    of _____ .

88. Heterosexual means _____ .

89. Lipoderm is _____ skin.

90. Neuralgia means _____ in a

    _____ .

91. Hematemesis means _____ .

92. Pyogenic means _____

93. Endocarditis means _____ of

    the_____ from within.

94. Cholelithiasis: condition of _____
    in bladder (gallbladder).

95. Phagocytosis means a condition of _____ .

96. Anodyne is _____ .

97. Microscope: an instrument to examine something _____

    _____ .

98. Telescope: an instrument to examine something _____

    _____ .

99. Atrophy is a lack of _____ .

100. Android means _____ man.

INDEX